Praise for Amy B. Sch

How to Heal Yourself When No

"[Amy Scher is] an inspiration, n
how to take healing into our ow
ing proof that it works."

—Pam Grout, #1 *New York Times* bestselling author of
E-Squared and *E-Cubed*

"Amy has seen the truth and can be a coach to all those who
seek healing and authenticity.... The potential resides in all of
us, so read on, do not fear failure, and fulfill your potential
while living an authentic life that you create and not one im-
posed by others."

—Bernie Siegel, MD, author of *A Book of Miracles* and
The Art of Healing

"Amy Scher has penned a remarkable book about the pivotal
role of the body, mind, and spirit in attaining true and complete
healing. There is much wisdom in this book, written with ex-
ceptional clarity, love, and wisdom."

—Sanjiv Chopra, MD, MACP, Professor of Medicine at
Harvard Medical School and bestselling coauthor
with Deepak Chopra of *Brotherhood*

"Amy Scher takes you on a guided journey to resolve emotional, physical, and energetic blockages that get in the way of true
healing. You will feel like you have a loving expert coach by
your side along the way."

—Heather Dane, coauthor with Louise Hay of
Loving Yourself to Great Health

"Amy Scher is a voice of calm, reassuring wisdom. Her own
triumph over illness is truly inspirational, but what really puts

Amy in an inspirational category of her own is her warm, kind, down-to-earth, truly accessible approach."

—Sara DiVello, bestselling author of *Where in the OM Am I?*

"Amy's story is awe-inspiring. Her book is full of wisdom and easy-to-implement techniques that have the power to help anyone reconnect their mind with their body and their heart with their soul and heal their entire lives. A really beautiful read."

—Luminita D. Saviuc, author of *15 Things You Should Give Up to Be Happy*

"*How to Heal Yourself When No One Else Can* is a comprehensive and user-friendly DIY manifesto that's the real deal. Amy guides readers toward authentic self-healing in a way that's easily accessible, honest, and relevant for today."

—Chris Grosso, author of *Indie Spiritualist*

"Amy is a courageous pioneer in the field of mind-body-spirit healing. With proven, easy-to-follow techniques, you will gain insight into the root cause of pain, physical dysfunction, and illness and transform your health.... This book illuminates the path to wellness."

—Sherrie Dillard, author of *Develop Your Medical Intuition*

This Is How I Save My Life
"Amy Scher is a brave warrior and a wonderful writer. She is a living example (very much living!) of what it looks like when a woman takes her health, her heart, and her destiny into her own hands. My hope is that this book will inspire many other women to do the same."

—Elizabeth Gilbert, #1 *New York Times* bestselling author of *Eat Pray Love* and *Big Magic*

How to
Heal Yourself
from Anxiety
*When No One
Else Can*

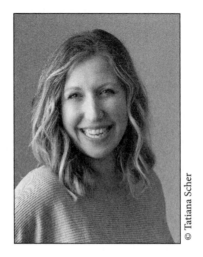

About the Author

Amy B. Scher is a bestselling author and a leading voice in the field of mind-body-spirit healing. As an energy therapist, Amy uses techniques to help those experiencing illness and those in need of emotional healing. She has been featured in the *Los Angeles Review of Books*, CNN, *Cosmopolitan*, CBS, the Huffington Post, and more. She was also named one of *The Advocate*'s "40 Under 40." Amy teaches and speaks internationally and is recognized for her inspirational story and approachable style. Her books have been translated into ten languages. She lives in New York City and can be found online at AmyBScher.com and YouTube.com/amybscher.

How to

Heal Yourself from Anxiety

When No One Else Can

AMY B. SCHER

Llewellyn Publications
Woodbury, Minnesota

First Edition
First Printing, 2019

Cover design by Shira Atakpu
Interior illustrations by Mary Ann Zapalac (all figurative art) and the
    Llewellyn Art Department

Llewellyn Publications is a registered trademark of Llewellyn Worldwide Ltd.

Library of Congress Cataloging-in-Publication Data
Names: Scher, Amy B., author.
Title: How to heal yourself from anxiety when no one else can / by Amy B.
    Scher.
Description: First edition. | Woodbury, Minnesota : Llewellyn Worldwide,
    [2019] | Includes index.
Identifiers: LCCN 2018046745 (print) | LCCN 2018049055 (ebook) | ISBN
    9780738756653 (ebook) | ISBN 9780738756462 (alk. paper)
Subjects: LCSH: Anxiety—Alternative treatment—Popular works.
Classification: LCC RC531 (ebook) | LCC RC531 .S26 2019 (print) | DDC
    616.85/22—dc23
LC record available at https://lccn.loc.gov/2018046745

Llewellyn Worldwide Ltd. does not participate in, endorse, or have any authority or responsibility concerning private business transactions between our authors and the public.

All mail addressed to the author is forwarded but the publisher cannot, unless specifically instructed by the author, give out an address or phone number.

Any internet references contained in this work are current at publication time, but the publisher cannot guarantee that a specific location will continue to be maintained. Please refer to the publisher's website for links to authors' websites and other sources.

Llewellyn Publications
A Division of Llewellyn Worldwide Ltd.
2143 Wooddale Drive
Woodbury, MN 55125-2989
www.llewellyn.com

Printed in the United States of America

Other Books by Amy B. Scher

How to Heal Yourself When No One Else Can
(Llewellyn, 2016)

*This Is How I Save My Life: From California to India,
a True Story of Finding Everything When You
Are Willing to Try Anything*
(Gallery Books, 2018)

*Llewellyn's Complete Book of Mindful Living:
Awareness & Meditation Practices for Living
in the Present Moment* (contributor)
(Llewellyn, 2016)

*Eat Pray Love Made Me Do It: Life Journeys Inspired by
the Bestselling Memoir* (contributor)
(Riverhead Books, 2016)

To my darling wife,
whose love and other superpowers
inspire me to be the best and calmest version
of myself—even when Mercury is in retrograde.
Which is pretty much all the time.
I love you beyond the beyond.

Acknowledgments

Thank you to my loving, amazing, entertaining family: You are everything to me. And especially to my mama, who never stops editing and laughing along with me.

Steve Harris, my literary agent: Thank you for continuing to be the most talented, kind, and cool agent there is. I will always be indebted to you for making all my publishing dreams come true.

To the team at Llewellyn: Angela Wix, my fabulous editor—thank you for helping to make every idea I have infinitely better. You are the best of the best. And to Andrea Neff, thanks to you for the crazy sprint to the finish line. This book wouldn't be what it is without you. Kat Sanborn, thank you for your enthusiasm and partnership in getting these pages into the hands of my beloved readers.

Sara DiVello: Still, always, and forever—together, we've got this.

To Nadine Nettman Semerau: Hallelujah for you and our constant texting! Writing shenanigans wouldn't be half as fun if you weren't just a beep away.

Kate Kerr-Clemenson: Every author needs "a Kate." I don't know how I got so lucky.

Contents

Exercises and Techniques

These are the exercises and techniques that you will learn throughout the book. Referring to this list will provide easy reference if you're looking for any one specific practice.

Images

This list will give you a reference point to easily find the visuals you need.

Disclaimer

The publisher and the author assume no liability for any injuries caused to the reader that may result from the reader's use of content contained in this publication and recommend common sense when contemplating the practices described in the work. This book and its practices are not a substitute for medical or psychiatric care.

Introduction

* * * * * * * * * * * * * * *

Essential Guidelines to Rock Your Healing

You have likely come to this book because you are feeling frustrated, scared, exasperated, and probably at your wits' end. Living with anxiety is no easy feat, but with this book in your hands, my intention is that your life is about to get not just easier but better. Lighter. Happier. It has been my life's work to help people just like you move from feeling anxious and helpless to feeling empowered, hopeful, and healed.

If you are familiar with my work, it may be because you have read my previous book *How to Heal Yourself When No One Else Can*, which shows readers how to use my unique approach to address a broad range of physical and emotional challenges. While you will find that the techniques and general approach in this book are similar, *How to Heal Yourself from Anxiety When No One Else Can* is laser-focused on addressing energetic blockages that are directly and specifically related to anxiety. The approach you will learn in these pages is targeted to *you*—a person who has tried everything and is still experiencing anxiety that prevents you from living life to the fullest.

It is important to work closely with your doctor in order to address all contributors to anxiety. While my approach is not a substitute for medical care, I have seen over and over that it can be an extremely beneficial complement to it and has often worked when other interventions have not. The gentle and effective process you will learn in this book will not interfere with any strategy employed by you and your medical practitioner. Addressing emotional imbalances in the energy system is an entirely different way of working to release anxiety, but you don't have to choose just one approach. You can do it all. My job, and the job of this book, is to help you understand and work with energetic factors that contribute to anxiety—factors that are not often addressed in other healing modalities.

Focus on the Big Picture

As I see it, anxiety is not *the* problem. Anxiety is the result of the real problem: unresolved emotional energies. The ultimate goal of all the work you will be doing is not to contain anxiety, learn to deal with it, or cope enough to simply get through your day. It is a much bigger picture: to truly address all the energetic causes of anxiety and release them for a happier, healthier, more relaxed and lighthearted *you*. It is to get you to feel as relaxed and safe in the world as possible, even when circumstances in life aren't perfect. This includes lightening up on yourself! I have never met a client who didn't have the pattern of being too hard on themselves, a tendency that contributes hugely to anxiety. Being easier on yourself will make a world of difference. All of the techniques we'll be using in this book will help you get to that finish line of feeling relaxed and safe—which is the *opposite* energy of anxiety. The two energies will not coexist.

If you are not leading the life that you thought you should or would, it doesn't mean you're broken. In fact, I see it as the exact opposite of that. When we are faced with a challenge like anxiety, we are forced to rise and meet it. It can even help us become who we were meant to be. That's what you are doing by working through my approach. You are breaking through, breaking free, breaking open in ways that could happen only by having your patience and persistence challenged. You are a total rock star! And as for the million-dollar question of "Why me?" my answer is that it doesn't matter. You are where you are for some reason that you might not fully understand. As someone who has been through this process and helped so many others through it too, I can assure you there is a bigger purpose that you may not have seen yet. *Yet.* But by showing up to do this healing work, you are helping yourself to realize it faster.

By keeping an eye on the ultimate goal of healing anxiety as a whole versus focusing only on how you can cope in the moment, you will be doing the work necessary to change your entire life.

Healing from anxiety is about using the place where you are now as an opportunity to let go of what is keeping you stuck. This practice will help you move closer and closer to the most lighthearted and relaxed version of yourself. When it seems like it's working, keep going. When it feels hard and seems like it's not working fast enough, do the same. Your new healing mantra is this: *Big picture, big picture, big picture, big picture.*

How This Book Will Help You

Most of the people I've worked with who have struggled with anxiety have been dealing with it for a long time and are often caught up in a detrimental pattern of blaming themselves for it. If this sounds like you, I'm here to help. This book is going to give you a wonderful new understanding of yourself and what you've been going through.

Again, anxiety is not the problem. Anxiety is also not simply just fear, like many people believe. Anxiety is the result of the *real* problem: unresolved emotional energies. Simply put, this is emotional baggage. What you will learn in the following pages will offer you not only a brand-new perspective but also an opportunity to follow a process of healing that may be very different from anything you've ever tried. Throughout the upcoming chapters I will be sharing a lot of insights and information about anxiety, and showing you exactly *how* to use that for your healing.

This book is not just about feeling better. This book will lay out my big-picture approach to healing the root of anxiety from an energetic perspective. We are going to cover a lot during our time together—but true healing comes from simply showing up for this work, slowly uncovering layers of emotional energy that are keeping you stuck, and consistently integrating what you learn into your life. You don't have to do every single thing in this book to successfully heal anxiety, and you don't have to do any of it perfectly. This process doesn't require you work on yourself for hours a day. I promise I'm going to make your journey as easy for you as possible.

You will learn how to release old emotional energy (aka emotional baggage) and the anxiety attached to it that your body has likely been holding on to for a long, long time. The process you are about to learn is a model that has been successful for me and for thousands of others through the client sessions and online programs that I've conducted.

Techniques in This Book

While there are many energy therapy techniques out there, many of them require special tools or another person to help you. All of the techniques you'll learn in this book will give you full power over your journey. You will not need to depend on anyone or anything but yourself to help you perform or practice them.

These are the main techniques you'll be learning:

- **Emotional Freedom Technique (EFT)**
- **Chakra Tapping**
- **Thymus Test and Tap (TTT)**
- **The Sweep**

With the exception of Emotional Freedom Technique (EFT), the main techniques in this book are ones that I created during my own healing journey and are now widely used all around the world. For each of the techniques I teach you, I'll offer suggestions to help you apply it directly to your own situation.

Outside of the four main techniques, you'll also be learning others that will help support you in your healing journey. A complete list of all the techniques and exercises can be found in the front of this book. The best way for me to teach you techniques is to explain the way that I use them for myself. However, please view these techniques and my explanations of them as loose guidelines, and feel free to revise and tweak them to fit what feels good to you. There isn't a single technique that I haven't altered or changed over the years as I've grown and learned. If you feel a nudge to change something, add to it, or revise it, you have my total permission to do that! When I was healing, I often made the following alterations: used a technique for a longer or shorter period of time than suggested, changed words or scripts to fit my specific situation, tapped for a different number of times than recommended, and so on.

The real secret to successful energy work has nothing to do with how perfectly you use these techniques. It's really about discovering *what* could be cleared and then being persistent in doing the work to clear it. In our work together I want you to be a curious detective about your own emotional energies, but try your best to be free from worrying about doing everything perfectly. It's much more important and effective to use the information you gather to do what you can, *when* you can, and in a way that feels right to you. You'll never be able to find and clear every single old energy, and that's okay too. Remember, we're looking at the big picture and trying our best to address things in each area outlined in this book for overall healing. That approach is more than enough. I want you to get to the healing in any way that works for you rather than being stalled by a fear of doing it "wrong."

How to Use This Book

Releasing anxiety using my approach is essentially a makeover for your entire energy system. We are going to be working on many different aspects of your healing to get you the best possible results. This book has been written in part as an exploratory process, in part as a how-to, and in part as a way to provide the insights and encouragement needed to keep you going when things feel hard. The real-life examples I share are from actual sessions in which my clients volunteered and/or gave me permission to tell their stories. Even so, each client's name and identifying details have been changed completely to fully protect their privacy.

The most effective way to go through this book and utilize my approach is to read, learn, and practice as you go along. I urge you to try things out, feel your way through them, and take action while you are immersed in each chapter. Each chapter is built on what you learned last, so going in order is the best way to really grasp and incorporate what you learn. Once in a while I'll hear from someone who says "I read your whole book and still don't feel good!" only to find out they haven't actually used the techniques. My approach can change your life only if you integrate it *into* your life.

Remember, our big-picture goal is to get you to feel as relaxed and safe in the world as possible, even when circumstances in life aren't perfect. Each page in this book will help you get to that main goal. I want to reassure you here that doing even just a little bit from each part of my approach can make a huge positive difference in how you feel.

Part 1: Calm and retrain your body

Part 2: Deal with your feelings

Part 3: Release stuck emotions

Part 4: Clear unprocessed experiences from the past

Part 5: Change harmful beliefs

You don't need to try to figure out all of your emotional baggage and fix it overnight. In fact, you couldn't even address every single stuck emotion, unprocessed experience, or harmful belief if you tried. We can never "get it all." That's okay. You can heal anyway. I am certainly not free of all emotional baggage, but I live a happy and healthy life anyway. I'm going to be guiding you to do the same.

Once you've read and made use of what you learned in each chapter in this book, you'll know my entire method. My healing approach is not a step-by-step process where you do one thing, check it off the list, and then move on to the next item. So let's talk about the very best way to make my approach work for you.

Where to Start for Your Healing

The first thing to know about where to begin the healing process is this: actually *starting* is the only thing that matters. It doesn't matter where you start when working on anxiety because you don't have to clear or release every single "negative" emotion, belief, or pattern from your life in order to heal from anxiety. You simply don't have to be perfect or do this work perfectly in order to be healthy and happy. Phew!

Also, the mind and the body are truly the *mind-body*. The two are so interconnected that it's almost impossible to focus on one aspect of anxiety without also unknowingly healing other parts of ourselves. This means that you are often doing even more positive work and getting more benefit than you realize.

For example, I had a client who experienced severe anxiety whenever he had to go to a store, even just to grab one item at the supermarket. This caused so many challenges that he became virtually housebound. The main goal of our work together was to get him to feel comfortable and relaxed when entering and being in a store. After several sessions he was delighted to find he could effortlessly go into any store and stay there for as long as he wanted. Within a couple months he got a great surprise: the regular headaches he got each morning upon waking started to lessen in intensity, and eventually they disappeared completely! Because one issue can be connected to many others, we are often doing more extensive clearing than we realize. When we cleared energies related to his anxiety, we obviously created a big shift in his relationship to the headaches too. Bonus!

That experience with my client is a perfect example of why we shouldn't get too caught up in exactly what order to do things in. Just keep chipping away at that rock from whatever angles you're led to. I want you to trust that everything you're working on—no matter how small it might seem—is part of the bigger picture of your healing.

What to Expect During the Healing Process

Starting a new healing process is exciting but can also cause some anxiety because it is all new. Knowing what to expect can help mitigate fear or doubt and expedite healing. Here are some important things to know.

How Long Will It Take to See Results?

While using the techniques in this book to release anxiety, you may feel relief right away or it may take persistence and time. Either one is fine. How fast you feel results doesn't matter at all to your overall success. Each of us is so unique, with different patterns, layers, and reactions to healing work. I know, I know—that might not be the answer you want. Healing is a process of gently working on layers of emotional stuff that has contributed to where you are today. It's a weaving, flowing process that we can't quite put a timeline on. I was so frustrated about this during my own healing process, but I soon learned that the body knows exactly at what pace and in what order it needs to release things.

I have found over and over again that when we just go with the flow, the healing happens. Sometimes seemingly small energies need to be released before we can get to the bigger layers that are keeping symptoms locked in place. Trust your intuition about where to go with using the tools and techniques from this book. Sometimes I see the greatest benefit when a client and I explore something that I never could have planned for. Sometimes things shift very quickly and sometimes the change is more subtle and gradual. If the anxiety you're experiencing has been long-standing, it's more likely to take a while of working at it from different angles to see a shift. Anxiety typically does not show up overnight, even though it might feel that way. That means it's unlikely to disappear overnight either. However,

I often see people have improvements in as soon as a few days to a few weeks. And miracles (or what I call "one-session wonders") do happen too, so be open to instant results.

Processing Old Energy Out of Your Body

When moving and releasing energy, people sometimes feel some "processing" occurring. This processing happens when your body releases the old energy completely from your energy field, which extends far beyond your physical body. The processing typically lasts for three to five days, although it can be longer for some people. During this time, it's possible you could temporarily feel subtly worse while your body lets go of the old and recalibrates itself. There is no need to worry about it though, as the processing phase is never permanent.

As you do this work more, you'll become attuned to your body's release process. I almost always see that if a person has a hard time in the beginning, it gets easier as their body adjusts to the clearing process. If processing is really rough for you, slow down and work in baby steps, get some extra rest, drink some extra water, and use the Ease Processing Discomfort tapping script in the appendix.

What Energy Therapy Feels Like

As you perform the techniques in this book, you might notice some signs that energy is moving, such as yawning, burping, getting the chills, hearing your stomach gurgle, sneezing, having a runny nose or eyes, or even feeling your emotions more intensely than before. All of these are good indicators that your body is releasing old emotional energy and things are moving. Yawning in particular is actually a signal that your nervous system is relaxing, and a relaxed nervous system puts you right in healing mode! If you feel nothing, that's perfectly okay too. I've had several clients who experienced no signs of energy releasing during the process but healed from anxiety anyway. I myself am a nonstop yawner! And once in a while, if I or my client is releasing a big amount of energy, I'll sneeze. I joke that my sneeze is worth ten yawns during a session. Just as everyone's healing pace is different, everyone's healing process is unique too.

How Much Time Should I Dedicate to Energy Work?

Because you are working on shifting old energetic patterns and retraining your system to be balanced and calm, consistency is key. Your body has likely been in a pattern of holding on for some time. The goal is to integrate these techniques into your life in order to retrain your body to let go instead. When I first started using energy therapy for my own healing, I set out to be organized and methodical in the process. That didn't last long! I soon learned two important lessons. First, dealing with emotions as you become aware of them on a day-to-day basis is essential for healing. (You'll learn about this in chapter 5.) If you imagine yourself as a pot of boiling water, you can understand why letting steam (emotions) out a bit at a time is better than waiting until you "have time to deal with them." Second, you need to dedicate separate time to do more in-depth work such as clearing emotional baggage from the past. (We'll cover this in section 3.) There is no set formula for how often to work on yourself or how long to work on each issue you find.

I suggest doing the following:

- Begin with the simple foundational practices you'll learn in chapter 1.
- Do the exercises from chapter 4 a few minutes each day to calm and retrain your system.

- Use techniques from chapter 5 to deal with your feelings daily, as needed.

- Do a few energy-clearing sessions each week to work with addressing the root of anxiety (from section 3).

The minutes you devote to this work on a *consistent* basis can change your life.

Do I Need to Keep Track of My Process?

I suggest that you keep a notebook dedicated to your emotional healing and jot down thoughts, ideas, or memories that come to mind as you learn. You may get insights into why you feel the way you do, when certain challenges began for you, or other ideas and clues about what you need to address. It can be useful to have a place to write down ideas you have about healing, subtle shifts you see in the anxiety, and observations you become aware of along the way. You will have a lot of ideas about what you need to release as you learn about the kinds of things that might be keeping you stuck. Simply note them in your journal. Clearing layers of emotional blocks is a marathon, not a sprint. Just keep an ongoing list so you always have something to chip away at.

How to Know If You're Making Progress

Together we will be working on anxiety using an energetic approach, and as this energy shifts, we will look for subtle signs of change. It's very typical for beginners or those wanting to feel better instantly (I certainly can't blame anyone for that!) to miss these signs. Signs of subtle healing include the following:

- feeling even one percent less anxious

- having a panic attack that lasts for a shorter amount of time than usual

- recovering more quickly from a spike in anxiety

- feeling more hopeful *about* the anxiety and your future in general

These are all indications that something is shifting internally.

Sometimes it may feel like nothing's improving and then suddenly all that great clearing you've been doing brings about change that you can really see and feel! For deep and permanent healing, there isn't always a quick fix. Healing typically doesn't happen in the way we imagine or want it to, but that doesn't mean it's not happening.

Now it's time to get started! I'm going to make this process as simple and rewarding as it can possibly be. By the end of our time together, you will not only understand why you've been struggling up until this point but also be well into the process of strengthening yourself to the core so you feel strong, balanced, and calm.

It's your time.

Section I

* * * * * * * * * * * * * * * *

My Approach to Healing Anxiety

* * * * * * * * * * * * * * *

Chapter One

Energy Therapy for Powerful Self-Healing

My approach to working with anxiety was born from my own experience of suffering from it and then healing myself. In this chapter, I will share with you my personal story of living with anxiety and my discoveries about the body's energy system and how it can be accessed for true healing. I will also introduce you to my self-created approach to healing anxiety, which has now helped people heal when nothing else has worked.

My Own Success Story with Energy Therapy

I was a happy, creative, outgoing kid who grew up in a family that fostered love, self-expression, and security. But I also had another side of me that was in deep contrast to that. It felt like I was always worried on the inside. I worried about things that other kids never seemed to give a thought to, like having to be away from my parents all day at school, failing a test, upsetting people, making a mistake, getting in a car accident, my mom and dad dying, and just about anything else you could think of. Beneath my happy-go-lucky little girl self, I had a persistent feeling of being on edge, always feeling like something bad was happening or going to happen. I felt like I was responsible for everything and everyone around me.

I was ten years old when my grandfather died, and then my dad almost simultaneously began to struggle with depression. But I never shared with anyone how that truly affected me. In fact, it had always been my natural pattern to keep my emotions tucked very deep inside. I didn't want to rock the boat or upset anyone. Instead, I strived to be the person who could handle anything. And a lot of the time I *was* actually that person. The problem was that I rarely allowed myself to fall apart, even when I really needed to.

It was in the years following my grandpa dying and my dad getting sick that things really started to shake me. I starting missing school a lot and getting sick all the time, and I felt anxious for no apparent reason. I saw many different types of doctors and therapists to help with all of it, and eventually was put on various antidepressants and anti-anxiety medications. By the time I graduated high school, I was *coping* with the anxiety, but only with medications, and the anxiety was still always there at some level.

In 2007, after being near death due to a mysterious illness that had been plaguing me for years, I was finally diagnosed with chronic, or late-stage, Lyme disease. This diagnosis only magnified the fears about life that I already had: *The world is unsafe. Something bad will happen. People get sick and die.*

It was during this stretch of time that I started to realize how much my pattern of emotional suppression was really affecting me. Anxiety had always been a big problem in my life, but being so physically sick made it impossible to run away from it for the first time ever.

Through my healing journey from chronic illness, I came to understand that anxiety had played an instrumental part in the manifestation of physical illness for me. Anxiety had been taking a toll on my body for years before any physical issues developed.

I always believed that anxiety was something that came out of nowhere and couldn't be controlled and that I would have to deal with it forever. And my perspective on anxiety only fueled my original fear of being unsafe.

It was only when I turned inward to address the emotional issues that had been plaguing me for much of my life that everything began to change and improve for me. It was in following this path that I discovered a shocking truth about anxiety. Anxiety is not a condition in and of itself but rather is a *side effect* of a dangerously unhealthy pattern that many humans, like myself, learn to perfect: suppressing emotions. Anxiety was my body's way of speaking to me, of alerting me to the fact that something wasn't right and I needed to pay attention. When I ignored that message that my body wasn't happy with my unhealthy emotional patterns, my body spoke through physical symptoms.

I realized that to heal permanently and completely, you must become who you really are; and you can't be *who* you really are when you're suppressing *how* you really feel.

This epiphany helped me approach healing from a brand-new angle—using energy therapy to access my stored emotions, work with my subconscious mind, and release deeply held patterns that I wasn't even aware of. By doing this, I healed myself from the inside out using the exact same process I am going to teach you in this book.

Emotions and the Body's Energy System

I grew up understanding my body as the physical mass that was a home for my organs, caused me grief as an awkward teenager, and made me clumsy in sports. But really, our bodies are so much more than we see. Everything in the universe (including human beings) is all just energy. We are made of an intricate energy system where electrical impulses run through us. These impulses have an effect on every part of our body: our organs, muscles, glands, and more. Every part of us interacts with this energy system, including our emotions, thoughts, and beliefs. In fact, our emotions are really just energy too!

It has long been known that our emotions are stored in the body at a cellular level. Candace Pert, PhD, author of *Molecules of Emotion*, was the person who opened my eyes to this. Dr. Pert's work is based on important findings about how feelings and unexpressed emotion from experiences can get stuck in the body. She explains that only when emotions are expressed can all the systems in the body be made whole—or, in other words, heal: "When emotions are repressed, denied, not allowed to be whatever they may be, our network pathways get blocked, stopping the flow of the vital feel-good, unifying chemicals that run both our biology and our behavior."[1]

Anxiety is not an evil entity trying to ruin your life or the product of an unhappy childhood; it is simply the messenger for emotions that need to be expressed in the body. Every human has emotions, which makes every human prone to anxiety.

I see the energy system as the overarching network that encompasses both the mind and the body, and energy therapy is a way "in" so we can access the emotions stored in our system and release them. Energy psychology, which is the basis of this book, is a group of energy therapy techniques that specifically address the relationship between the energy system and emotions, thoughts, and behavior. By using energy therapy in this

---

1. Candace B. Pert, PhD, *Molecules of Emotion: Why You Feel the Way You Feel* (New York: Scribner, 1997), 273.

way, we can release the related emotional energies contributing to the anxiety. No more "just coping."

You may be familiar with the concept of energy in the body and not even know it! Modern diagnostic medical tools such as EEGs (which measure brain waves) and EKGs (which measure the electrical activity of the heart) are essentially measuring a type of energy. This technology has been around for a long time, but there is another type of energy that is not yet detectable with most modern tools. This type of energy is often referred to as "subtle energy." This subtle energy has been seen and felt by healers and energy-sensitive people for thousands of years. Traditional Chinese Medicine and Ayurveda, both ancient medical systems, are based on addressing the body's subtle energies. Subtle energies are what we'll be working with throughout this book. Everything that affects you is connected to this energy system. You can think of it as the foundation or core of your being. And by working with this system, you can change everything in its field. The energy system helps you access the emotions that have been keeping you stuck and let them out.

Within the body's main subtle energy system are various parts (or subsystems): chakras, meridians, auras, and more. Throughout this book, we will work directly with meridians and chakras. However, because all of the parts of your energy system work together, we will be affecting and strengthening all of it.

A Brief Overview of Meridians and Chakras

Later in this book you'll be learning how to work with two major parts of your energy system: meridians and chakras. Here is a brief overview to get you acquainted with these amazing parts of your body system.

Meridians

These are energy highways that flow throughout your entire body and deliver energy to everything along each specific pathway: organs, glands, muscle, and more. Each meridian has its own name, is associated with a specific function in the body, and relates to specific emotions. You'll learn more about meridians in chapter 5 when you learn Emotional Freedom Technique (EFT).

There is one specific meridian—called the *triple warmer meridian*—that is so powerful and important to your mental and physical health that it acts as its own energy subsystem. The triple warmer meridian governs what's called the *fight, flight, or freeze response* in the body, which I like to refer to as the body's "freak-out mode." You'll be learning more about the triple warmer meridian and how to work with it in chapter 4.

Chakras

The chakras are spinning energy centers in the body that hold the energies of old stories and imprints from our lives. Each chakra covers a specific part of the body, correlates with specific emotions, and affects the physical area of the body where it is located. You'll learn more about chakras in chapter 5 when you learn a technique called *Chakra Tapping*.

Symptoms, both emotional and physical, are created when our energies are disrupted, flow irregularly, or become sluggish and blocked. Even if your primary challenge is anxiety, the energy imbalances that may be contributing to it can often still be felt in the body. An energy imbalance in your system can feel like a knot in the pit of your stomach, burning in your chest, or tension in your back or neck. These types of symptoms are indications that you are experiencing a lack of energy flow to those specific areas because of stuck emotional energy. That is what an imbalance is.

There are many things that interact with and negatively affect our energy system, such as the foods we eat, environmental toxins, and where we live and work. However, in my experience, emotional energies often have a greater impact on us than these types of external factors. In fact, releasing stuck emotional energy can help strengthen the entire body, making us less likely to react adversely to other things. In order to rebalance the body's energy system, we need to release the emotions stored within it.

Different energetic approaches and healing systems may address only specific parts of the overall energy system. For example, we'll be focusing primarily on meridians and chakras. But remember, because all the subsystems work together, your entire system will benefit.

Jan's story is a great example. Jan's doctor sent her to me because she'd had several blood tests indicating that her liver enzymes were elevated. They couldn't figure out why or what to do with them. For many years Jan had struggled with anxiety, which was partially under control with meds, but recently it had really kicked up again. Her doctor suspected that these symptoms were all linked together. Jan and I worked on identifying and clearing emotional energies from her past that were stuck in her body, just like you'll learn to do in section 3. It was a few weeks before the levels of both her anxiety and her liver enzymes decreased dramatically. During the time we were working together, she changed nothing else. We discovered that the anxiety spike had been caused by emotions stuck in her body, specifically in the area of her liver. When we used energy therapy to release the emotions causing blockages in her energy system, the energy flow returned to her liver, and it was able to function properly again.

If you have exhausted all the mainstream options for dealing with anxiety, like I did, I think you'll find my approach refreshing and eye-opening. I hope it will give you a whole new way to understand anxiety, show you that you have more power than you might believe, and help you to improve your life. The coolest part is that working with your energy system is free and effective and has no negative side effects. And it won't interfere with any current treatment plan that you and your doctor already have in place.

Why Energy Therapy Is So Beneficial

If you're anything like I used to be, you might feel like self-healing comes with a lot of pressure. Maybe it feels impossible to imagine how you will ever get to a place of feeling calm, relaxed, and balanced when you're struggling so much right now. But let me explain why and how it totally *is* possible.

One of the absolute biggest contributors to anxiety is the feeling of being unsafe in this world, which sets off the fight, flight, or freeze response in the body. Self-healing immediately works on counteracting that deep-seated feeling with every application. In essence, it reverses the feeling of helplessness. By using self-healing, you will be affirming the messages of "I can be okay no matter what" and "I can help myself!" These two messages are essential for healing anxiety. They will help you feel safe in your own hands. Owning your healing process in this way helps bolster your own sense of safety and capability and actually eliminates some of what triggers anxiety in the first place. In other words, the practice of self-healing acts as its own anti-anxiety modality, regardless of what techniques or practices you use. This is such an incredible added benefit of doing this work! Throughout the process that we'll follow in this book, you will come to realize that you are a part of the solution to a problem that you have felt wildly out of control of.

The only requirement for healing is that we need to do our part to clear emotions, beliefs, and patterns that no longer work for us. These are the energies that are speaking to us through the anxiety. Our job is to listen and address our body's messages. The rest will unfold from there. Even while getting the support of medications and therapies that we might already be pursuing, we cannot excuse ourselves from doing the inner work if we truly want to be free from anxiety. We need to identify and release the long-held emotional patterns stored inside of us. In order to put anxiety out of its job, we need to help our body chill out, relax, and embrace the message that we are safe.

An Introduction to My Approach

There are five main parts to work toward with my approach to ensure we are addressing all the energetic components of anxiety. They don't all need to be done at the same time and they don't all need to be done perfectly and completely, but we want to keep all five in mind for the best healing results.

Part 1: Calm and Retrain Your Body

If you've been experiencing anxiety, your body has likely been in the bad habit of being in freak-out mode. This state of being is often referred to as the fight, flight, or freeze response, wherein your body responds to stress in one of the following ways: *fights* its way through (or out of) stress, takes *flight* or tries to flee from stress, or *freezes* in order to cope with stress. When you experience difficult emotions or physical or emotional trauma, the fight, flight, or freeze response is triggered in your system temporarily. This is a healthy response to stress that helps you survive it. However, if you store emotional energies related to the trauma in your body long after the event that caused the stress, you can actually get stuck in this freak-out state.

The fight, flight, or freeze response is governed by the triple warmer meridian, an energetic dynamic that is an important part of the body's overall energy system and is closely tied to anxiety. It is also linked to patterns of self-sabotage, which can prevent you from taking even the tiniest step in the right direction. You'll learn more about the triple warmer meridian and the fight, flight, or freeze response in chapter 4. Calming your body and training it to move out of freak-out mode and into chill-out mode is essential to any successful healing program for anxiety. You will be guided to learn exactly how to do this.

Part 2: Deal With Your Feelings

Because it feels so bad to be anxious, we often avoid truly dealing with it. But *not* dealing with our feelings is part of the reason anxiety develops in the first place, so creating a new pattern of addressing our feelings must come before we even attempt to figure out why, when, and how the anxiety started in the first place. I am going to give you tools you can use to deal with your feelings and become empowered—now. You will be learning two great techniques, Emotional Freedom Technique (EFT) and Chakra Tapping. These will help you begin to release and neutralize any uncomfortable feelings you have right now and allow you to dig deeper into the root causes and triggers of anxiety.

Part 3: Release Stuck Emotions

Suppressed emotions from the past that end up stuck in the body can contribute to anxiety in two ways. First, emotions that are not felt and processed throughout your life become stuck inside of you, causing you to feel those emotions at some level all the time, sometimes even just subconsciously. Second, having old emotions lodged in your system creates anxiety be-cause those suppressed emotions are trying to bubble up and break free. In addition, having emotions such as fear, anger, and resentment stuck in your body can trigger the triple warmer meridian (which, as a reminder, governs your fight, flight, or freeze response) to go into overdrive, which sets off the freak-out response in your body. This can cause you to feel on edge or unsafe in addition to the original emotions that you are still feeling. Most approaches to anxiety relief teach you how to cope with these emotions, but in our work together you are going to actually release stuck emotions from your body com-pletely. I will provide detailed instructions on exactly how to do just that.

Part 4: Release Unprocessed Experiences from the Past
Any disturbing or distressing event or emotional experience from your past that you have not properly moved out of your body may still be affecting you today. You'll learn how to deal with memories that are negatively affecting you, which I call *unprocessed experiences*. Releasing these unprocessed experi-ences will help eliminate triggering memories from your sys-tem—a huge part of your healing.

Part 5: Clear Harmful Beliefs
Ideas or messages that we learn early in life become the beliefs we live our lives by. Oftentimes, these beliefs are running on au-topilot in the subconscious mind. However, our beliefs are not fact. Believing things like the world is unsafe or we have to be perfect in order to be loved contributes to anxiety. These beliefs magnify the body's freak-out response. On the flip side, some-times our subconscious mind will believe that anxiety protects us and that we actually need it. This is something I see in every

client I work with. No matter what kinds of beliefs you have or how many there are (and there may be a lot!), we'll be going through the very easy but effective process of clearing them.

Are you starting to get a sense of why you feel so yucky and overwhelmed? Deep and permanent healing comes from getting your whole self to relax into life so you can be who you really are and live freely.

Now that you know exactly what kind of healing adventure you're in for, it's time to dig deeper into anxiety and begin to let it go completely.

Create a Solid Healing Foundation

I'm going to teach you how to use a few quick energy-balancing exercises to create a solid foundation for your healing. Think of these as laying the groundwork for the deeper work you'll be doing in the coming chapters. If you are able to spend two to five minutes on each of these, once in the morning and then again in the evening, you'll be golden! But just do whatever you can.

Grounding

Grounding (sometimes called *earthing*) is the practice of connecting yourself to the earth's north and south poles. When you do this, it allows the natural healing properties and rhythms of the earth to rectify the effects of the polarity reversal. Throughout history, humans have walked barefoot and slept on the ground. This process helped the body calibrate itself to the electrical rhythm of the earth, stabilizing the electrical current of organs, tissues, and cells. In other words, our bodies worked with full battery power because our polarities were functioning correctly.

The process of grounding very gently affects the triple warmer energy dynamic. Research has shown that after grounding, subjects experience a decrease in stress levels and a balancing of the autonomic nervous system (again, the primary system involved in the fight, flight, or freeze response).

How to Ground: The best and easiest way to ground is to simply put your feet on the dirt, sand, grass, or unsealed concrete. Then just hang out for a few minutes. The longer you practice grounding, the more benefit you will receive, so feel free to grab a book to read and extend your time as long as you can. It's that easy. If you aren't able to be outside, I suggest bringing in some "earth" (rocks, dirt, etc.) and putting your feet in a big bowl or pot along with it.

Eye Trace

Energy is supposed to flow in a crossover pattern in the body. This is the body's natural pattern. There are many natural crossover patterns that are inherent in the body: the brain uses both the left and the right hemisphere together, our arms swing across our body when we walk, we crawl in a crossover direction when we are young, and even the shape of our DNA is a crossover pattern.

If your energy system has gotten out of this crossover pattern, it will begin to flow in an up-and-down pattern instead. This is what energy pioneer Donna Eden calls a "homolateral" energy flow in her popular book *Energy Medicine*.[2] When your energy is running in this homolateral pattern, you are not functioning at your full healing capacity. In my experience, this homolateral flow has a very negative effect on our emotions and thoughts, creating a feeling of being scrambled, stressed, and

2. Donna Eden, with David Feinstein, *Energy Medicine: How to Use Your Body's Energies for Optimum Health and Vitality* (London: Piatkus, 1999).

out of control. That's why it's essential to correct this flow when dealing with anxiety.

Luckily, the correction for homolateral energy is easy—as long as you are persistent. And if you happen to be the rare person with anxiety whose energy is already flowing in a crossover pattern, this exercise won't hurt you.

Attaining and maintaining the crossover pattern in the body is essential to getting yourself to a place of healing. To help encourage your energies to cross over, you can simply trace in a crossover pattern around the eyes. When working to overcome anxiety, this can be done for a couple minutes a few times a day. But again, if you forget or don't hit your goal each day, don't worry. A little goes a long way.

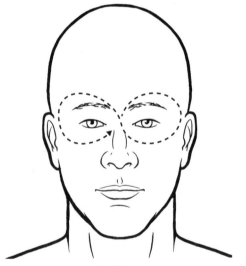

Eye Trace

Thymus Tapping

The thymus gland is the master gland of the body's immune system and is located in the upper part of the chest, behind the breastbone. It sits right over the heart. The thymus is responsible for making T-cells, which are vital to the healthy functioning of the immune system, providing protection against allergies, autoimmune diseases, and immunodeficiency. The thymus gland is connected to the entire energy system and is so powerful that it can work as a stress modulator when stimulated.

A lot of people are naturally drawn to the thymus area when they are feeling anxious and don't even realize that their body is trying to help them tend to this special gland. Do you ever "flutter" your chest with your hands when you're upset? Think of how gorillas in the wild thump their chests if they perceive danger. In both these cases, it's a natural tendency to strengthen and balance our energy when we need it most. See, you're already doing this by accident! Now we're going to help you do it on purpose, too.

How to Tap the Thymus: Tapping the thymus gland using your fingertips is a powerful calming, strengthening, and balancing technique. I use it many times throughout the day. Simply tap with medium pressure while you breathe deeply. As an alternative, my favorite twist on this calming technique is to gently tap the thymus in a specific 1-2-3 rhythm to mimic a heartbeat. I use a flat hand against my chest for this, tapping my fingers against my thymus with the third "beat" or tapping with slightly firmer pressure than the rest. Tapping the thymus is both stimulating to the immune system and calming to the body at the same time.

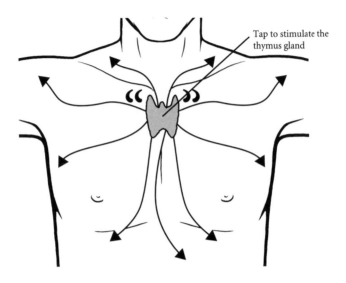

Tap to stimulate the thymus gland

Thymus Tapping

Note: Your thymus gland might be tender when you tap. Do not stop because of this. Tenderness is usually a sign that there is some stagnant energy there, which means you really need to do this exercise. Over time, as your thymus becomes more balanced, it will become less sore.

Summary

Anxiety is a dynamic that plays out not only in the mind and the physical body but in the energy body too. Anxiety is simply a messenger for the body about emotions that need to be expressed and old energetic patterns that need to be changed. My approach to healing utilizes energy therapy, a gentle and effective way to access and release emotional energies contributing to anxiety. By working with your energies, the act of self-healing becomes its own modality, reversing a feeling of helplessness and restoring balance and calm.

My approach to healing anxiety is a complete system with five parts: calming and retraining your body, dealing with your feelings, releasing stuck emotions, clearing unprocessed experiences from the past, and changing harmful beliefs.

Chapter Two

* * * * * * * * * * * * * *

The Truth about Anxiety

Anxiety does not come from out of the blue. That's not how it works at all. In this chapter I will be sharing all of the truths I've learned about anxiety to help you understand it more completely, including outlining the origin of it and explaining how the subconscious mind can make it difficult (though not impossible at all!) to overcome. I know this will open your eyes to how you might have arrived in this place of feeling anxious and afraid in the first place, which will help you get to the next step: moving forward.

The Cause of Anxiety

I always saw anxiety as a condition that appeared out of nowhere, a force that I couldn't control, and thought I would have to cope with it for the rest of my life. It was only through my own healing that I discovered anxiety was very different from what I believed it to be.

When I start working with a client, they are often most concerned with what caused the anxiety in the first place. "I can't remember anything so bad in my life that I should have anxiety like this!" they tell me. But the truth is that anxiety does not usually have one cause. Anxiety is not a mysterious condition that pops up suddenly when everything is going perfectly in life, but rather is a *side effect* of a long-standing unhealthy pattern of ignoring or suppressing emotions that need to be addressed. The anxiety you are experiencing likely didn't come out of nowhere, although it certainly might seem like it. Anxiety can show up suddenly, but the imbalances related to it have likely been brewing in your energy system for a long time.

It's essential to understand that anxiety is not a single emotion; it's a dynamic that affects your entire system. Let's dig into some truths about anxiety so we can understand, unravel, and heal it—for a happier, more relaxed you.

What Is Anxiety?

There are many words we might use to describe how anxiety makes us feel: uncomfortable, scared, unsettled, conflicted, anxious, antsy, nervous, attacked, unsafe, and out of control. But there is one thing that almost everyone can agree on: it feels bad. In fact, anxiety is often described to me as a deep-seated feeling that something bad is happening or is about to happen. And this is actually quite accurate because something bad *is* happening—inside of you. Your body is feeling the imbalances that come from unresolved emotional energy, or baggage, in your system.

Anxiety comes from your body being in freak-out mode, not because of what's happening outside of you but because of what's stuck *inside of you*. While external circumstances outside of your control certainly may trigger you, that is not the actual origin of anxiety.

The feeling of anxiety arises because your body is trying so hard to keep old emotional baggage contained, and it's just too much for anyone to hold. Anxiety manifests when stored emotional energy is trying to bubble up and out. As I mentioned earlier, anxiety is not simply caused by fear. Anxiety can be caused by any emotional baggage that you have not dealt with. I've seen as many people with anxiety due to suppressed anger and frustration as due to fear. But I don't want you to be scared that every time you experience stress or strong emotions, you'll create emotional baggage that will cause a problem for you in the future. That's the whole point of all the work we're doing— to release old energies and patterns so you can deal with emotions in a healthier way going forward. We're going to bring your body into a calm and balanced state so your system can better handle both internal stress and the world around you.

How Anxiety Shows Up in Your Life

Now you understand that anxiety is not simply feeling panicked all the time or having fears and phobias. In fact, many people have anxiety and yet have absolutely none of the typical symptoms you might imagine. Anxiety can manifest in ways you may not even be aware of, including the following:

- Negative, compulsive, or obsessive thoughts
- Needing to be in control of life and others
- Inability to relax
- Difficulty making decisions
- Being too hard on yourself (self-critical)
- Resistance to accepting the help of others
- Feeling shaky or unstable
- Feeling sad, angry, or pretty much any other difficult emotion
- Being moody
- Inability to concentrate
- Digestive upset

- Heartburn

- Fatigue

- Sensitivity to lights, electromagnetic fields (EMFs), etc.

- Physical symptoms

I want to give you a few real-life examples so you can understand this better. All of these clients came to me with different challenges, but when we focused specifically on emotional energies related to anxiety, their lives and health improved tremendously. For each client, after they learned how to deal with their feelings coming up day to day (chapter 5), we worked with addressing the root of anxiety from section 3:

- Releasing stuck emotions (chapter 6)

- Clearing unprocessed experiences from the past (chapter 7)

- Changing harmful beliefs (chapter 8)

Sheryl had a racing heart and had felt on edge her whole life. She described it to me as feeling like she had just finished exercising—all the time. Any physical activity made this worse though, so she was unable to do any activity that might increase her heart rate. She had been from doctor to doctor with no relief. When Sheryl and I began working together, we started simply by helping her incorporate EFT into her life to deal with her feelings on a day-to-day basis. We then released stuck emotions that she had been carrying for most of her life. We were able to clear some unprocessed experiences (memories) from her past as well. We also worked on clearing the belief that "if I relax, something bad will happen." These few emotional blocks were so big that it was only about a week before she started feeling significantly better. "It feels like my heart slowed down fifty beats a minute!" she told me in an email, and joked that now she felt obligated to start exercising.

Tom, another client of mine, had such a sensitivity to lights that he could hardly leave his house. His body essentially went into freak-out mode every time he was around natural or synthetic lighting. He would get a headache, be overcome by a sense of panic, and have to lie down almost immediately. We released emotions stuck in his body that were being triggered by lights and also worked on the belief that "it's dangerous to be in the light," which was symbolic of his fear of attention. There were other similar energies we worked on over a period of four months, and now Tom can go anywhere with no problem at all.

Another client, Dan, had social anxiety that made it hard for him to have even a casual conversation with people he knew. He never realized that social anxiety was triggering generalized anxiety, even when he was home alone. In the back of his head, he was always worried about when he'd next have to talk to someone or interact with a group. We released stuck emotions from times in his past when talking to someone had made him feel embarrassed. We also released the belief that "people will pick on me when I talk to them." Over the next couple months, we continued clearing old energies from different parts of my approach. Dan now describes himself as a newly emerged social butterfly!

Essentially, we worked a little bit with each of the parts of my approach. You won't need to cover everything in order to see improvement, but over time, it's beneficial to address as much as you can from each part for the best results.

Anyone Can Be Affected by Anxiety

Anxiety can affect anyone, but many people believe that only weak or highly emotional people get anxiety. People who experience anxiety often feel bad about themselves, feeling delicate and unable to handle life in the way that others can. Sometimes these perceptions do actually become beliefs that perpetuate anxiety. Imagine subconsciously telling yourself all day, "I can't handle life" or "I'm so delicate." But nothing could be further from the truth.

Many people who experience anxiety have a constitutional makeup or personality traits that actually tend *toward* anxiety, such as being highly empathic, overachieving, self-sacrificing, or self-critical, or always being the "strong" one or a Type-A perfectionist who prides themselves on keeping everything under control.

Anxiety sufferers are often in leadership and caretaking roles and are able to "do or conquer anything." These are awesome personality traits to have. However, these people may also take on the world at the expense of themselves.

Anxiety May Not Even Be All Yours

While people with anxiety are not weak, it *is* actually quite true that those who struggle with anxiety may be "sensitive," though not in the way most people think. Those who experience anxiety are often highly attuned to the needs of others and sensitive to the energies of those around them. I call this dynamic "energetic sensitivity," meaning this person's own sense of safety and balance becomes compromised, often subconsciously, by taking on other people's energies. In other words, an energetically sensitive person can be a sponge for what's going on around them, and the anxiety they are feeling can actually come from picking up on other people's "stuff." Strengthening the body's energy system by releasing old emotional baggage (as we'll be doing throughout this book) is the best protection against being energetically sensitive. As you strengthen your core self, you will be less shaken by the world and the people around you.

In addition to being energetically sensitive, there is another explanation for why the anxiety you are experiencing may not be all yours. *Inherited* energies (sometimes called *generational* energies) are energies you inherited from your parents and ancestors. In the same way we inherit genes or personality traits, we can inherit unresolved emotional energy too. This is very common and I see it with almost every client I work with. People who are being affected by inherited energy often describe feeling like there has been a cloud over their head their whole life, and they often see the same anxiety patterns throughout their entire family as well. If you have inherited energy that's linked to anxiety, you may feel confused or detached from it, perhaps because it didn't originate from your own body in the first place. You'll be learning more about inherited energy and how to address it in chapter 10.

Why Healing Anxiety Can Be So Difficult to Overcome

Your subconscious mind can be your best friend and your biggest foe. Even without knowing you, I'm willing to bet that at this moment your subconscious mind is causing you a whole lot of trouble. Let me explain why, because understanding the subconscious mind is often the key to unraveling and healing anxiety.

There is an entire separate part of your being that's the real "boss" of your life: the subconscious mind. According to the biologist Bruce Lipton, PhD, the subconscious mind controls up to 95 percent of our lives. That includes decisions, emotions, actions, and behavior. Only 5 percent of our memories and other data reside in the conscious mind. The subconscious mind is the tape recorder of everything that's ever happened in our lives, including memories of events, emotions we've felt, and messages we've received from others. The subconscious mind then uses the data or programming it has from the past to make "rules" to live by for the future. These rules dictate much of our behavior and how we relate and respond to the world.

The subconscious mind will do anything to protect us or do what it thinks is *good* for us, according to its rules or programming. In terms of neurological processing tasks, the subconscious mind is more than a million times more powerful than the conscious mind. Thanks to our subconscious mind, which is always running on autopilot, we don't have to think about every bodily function or every task we do. But when the programming and the rules within the subconscious mind are actually triggering anxiety instead of helping us overcome it, it can be a problem. Because of how powerful the subconscious mind is, it can be very difficult to overcome anxiety unless we learn to work with the subconscious as our trusted friend and healing partner.

In each of the chapters in section 3, you'll be learning ways that you can work with your subconscious mind to transform this old programming and release anxiety. Woohoo! This is gonna be a game-changer for you.

Why You Can't "Just Get Over It"

Many anxiety sufferers are told that it's all in their head and they should just get over it. It's not hard to end up feeling like anxiety is your fault, that if only you had more willpower or discipline you could fix this. But, of course, it's not nearly that easy. One of the reasons it's impossible to take that approach is because, as you've just learned, your subconscious mind has likely been preventing you from overcoming it.

Let's look at some reasons that make the "just get over it" argument obsolete. Ready? Your guilt trip is about to end!

This is likely the complex process going on in your energy system right now, making it difficult for you to move forward.

Your Body Is Stuck in Freak-Out Mode: When your body is stuck in fight, flight, or freeze—or what I call freak-out mode—it's very difficult to heal. This freak-out mode is linked to the triple warmer meridian, which governs the fight, flight, or freeze response in the body. It affects the nervous system, immune system, and so much more. This freak-out response essentially creates a feeling of danger in your whole system. Anxiety is not just in your head; it's in your entire body. In order to fully heal, you need to calm and retrain your body to be relaxed and calm. In other words, you need to get your body out of freak-out mode and into healing mode. This is the entire focus of our work in chapter 4.

You Have Stuck Emotions in Your System: Emotions that you felt in the past can get lodged in the body. When they become stuck, you are essentially feeling each of those emotions (which can number in the hundreds or thousands) at a low level all the time. So it's no surprise now why you're feeling so uncomfortable, right? In addition, the sheer force of having to "hold" all of these unexpressed emotions can create a sense of anxiety. Releasing these emotions from the body is what we will be addressing in chapter 6.

Part of You May Believe That You Need Anxiety: The subconscious mind may not only know which emotions are stuck in your body (which you aren't consciously aware of) but is also likely using anxiety to protect you. While this may seem totally counterintuitive, anxiety is often created by the subconscious mind in order to feel safe. Anxiety is a state of being that your subconscious mind may feel keeps you on high alert and helps you stay "in control." This state often creates a false sense of safety. The subconscious mind may also use anxiety as a tool to protect you from dealing with something that it believes is even *worse* than anxiety. For example, your subconscious mind may perceive that feeling anxiety is better than having to deal with your true feelings or is easier than having to say no to people you love. We will be identifying and releasing the beliefs that your body has about why it *needs* anxiety in chapter 8.

Why You Shouldn't Even Try to "Just Get Over It"

"Be stronger than anxiety." "Use your willpower." "It's mind over matter." These are some of the things my clients tell me their friends and family suggest to them in order to speed up the healing process. Making a conscious choice that you are ready to heal from anxiety is necessary and healthy, but pushing yourself to "just get over it" could actually make it significantly worse.

The fact is, radical change—even change that's for the better—can cause great resistance within the body, triggering further anxiety.

It is important to know that while your body is in freak-out (or fight, flight, or freeze) mode, it will likely resist any change at all, especially if forced or pushed. When we try to change the pattern too quickly, the triple warmer meridian (which governs the fight, flight, or freeze response) can actually kick into high gear, creating even more anxiety. This meridian also governs habits. When the triple warmer meridian is on high alert, it will fight against all change in an effort to keep us safe. This is one reason why it can be so darn difficult to change a bad habit or create a healthier new one when we are in a stressed state. We often find ourselves resisting help, feeling overwhelmed (the triple warmer meridian is the king of overwhelm!), rebelling against things we know are good for us, and abandoning self-care. This is because our triple warmer meridian's resistance to change is acting as a form of self-sabotage, perceiving anything new or different as more dangerous or stressful than staying stuck where we are.

We already talked a bit about how beliefs can cause us to perceive (even if just at a subconscious level) that anxiety keeps us safe. Because we often have a deep-seated feeling of being unsafe, pushing to overcome our anxiety—which is likely to cause stress and more anxiety—can backfire and strengthen these types of beliefs. The body may actually feel *less* safe than it did before we tried to clear the anxiety.

Since you now understand that anxiety is often linked to the subconscious mind, you can see why using the conscious mind alone to "just get over it" is a pretty flawed plan. We really need to work with both the conscious *and* the subconscious mind in order to be fully empowered.

The initial step is going to be calming and retraining your body by addressing the fight, flight, or freeze response so you can get some relief and start sending a message to your entire system that it's safe to relax and begin to move forward now.

Let's go.

Summary

Anxiety is not a condition that comes from out of the blue to attack weak or delicate people. It may seem to show up suddenly, but the energetic imbalances in the body that helped to create it have likely been there for a long time.

Anxiety can show up in many subtle or obvious ways (including physical symptoms) that you might never have even recognized as anxiety. Because the subconscious mind is so powerful and is linked to the causes of anxiety, pushing to "just get over it" can actually cause the anxiety to become even stronger.

To fully overcome our anxiety, we need to work at it by gently calming the body's fight, flight, or freeze response and using the subconscious mind to determine what helped to create the anxiety in the first place.

Chapter Three

* * * * * * * * * * * * * * *

The Role of Your Subconscious Mind

Where did this anxiety come from? Why does it only get worse the more I try to make it better? What is triggering it? What would you say if I told you that you already have these answers you've been searching for? Well, it's true. You just haven't been able to access them yet. Here's why.

The part of you that's really in control of your life is your subconscious mind. The subconscious is like a human computer, recording everything that we've ever experienced—memories, messages, feelings, perceptions, and events from our lives. Because of this, so much of what we need to know in order to heal anxiety is locked in the subconscious.

In this chapter you'll learn about how the subconscious mind is programmed, what we can discover by tapping into that reservoir of information, and exactly how we can do that using a technique called *muscle testing* (sometimes called *energy testing* or *kinesiology*). This was an absolute game-changer for my own healing, and I trust that it can be for yours too.

The Hidden Information in the Subconscious Mind

The subconscious mind doesn't analyze or reason. It gathers data and stores it. Based on that stored data, it creates programming. Countless interpretations of experiences from childhood become the messages, beliefs, and perceptions that the subconscious mind uses to direct our behavior in life. Based on the data it has collected, primarily during childhood (up to the age of seven), the subconscious mind makes "rules" to live by and directs our behavior according to those rules. It's a little scary to consider that we make most of our decisions with the part of our mind that has the least information, acts like a seven-year-old, and is largely inaccessible to us. In kid terms, our subconscious mind is *the boss of us!* And up until now, it's likely that you haven't had any way of changing that for your healing. Yikes! You can see the potential mess here.

The dynamic I just described with the subconscious mind causes two very big challenges for us.

First, data that could be very useful to our healing is probably stuck in our subconscious mind. Some of this information includes the things we can release in order to heal more efficiently and completely. But how can we release them when we don't know what they are? We likely can recall only a small percentage of the experiences that our subconscious knows about. And as we talked about earlier, our conscious, rational mind might not be the best part of our brain to help us figure out what to work on (or else we wouldn't be where we are today).

Second, what if the rules and the programming of the subconscious mind are not actually beneficial for us? It's amazing how our subconscious mind functions on autopilot so much of the time, allowing us to go to the bathroom, write, or do so many other tasks without any thought at all. The subconscious mind is more than a million times more powerful than the conscious mind in terms of neurological processing, but what if the ideas that are stuck in the subconscious are hindering our life? As we keep going back to those memories, experiences, and interpretations of the past, we create new cells along those neural pathways, reinforcing old response patterns that may be contributing to anxiety. It can become a vicious cycle.

Hopefully you're laughing and not crying right now. If you're crying, don't worry. The good news is that when I help you tap into your subconscious mind, you will finally discover why you've been full of anxiety and stuck for so long, and you'll have brand-new information that will help you get unstuck and move on.

Why What's in Your Subconscious Mind Matters

Tapping into your subconscious mind can be a big piece of your healing because if you're not aware of what's in there, you can't release it or change it. And if you're anything like I used to be or like most of my clients are, you have no idea what's *really* causing the anxiety or keeping you in the anxiety loop. If you did, then addressing the things you thought were causing anxiety would be making a difference for you.

The subconscious mind can make it easier to identify the causes of anxiety and can help you overcome it by aligning with your healing. Here's how.

Use the Subconscious Mind to Help Identify the Causes of Anxiety

You might have some memories that you've connected to the anxiety that you've been dealing with for months or maybe even years. Maybe you remember a particular event in your life, such as a time when you were really scared because you were left home alone. And while an event like that could possibly be a contributing factor, that memory might also feel connected for you because it makes sense to your logical mind. Being alone = fear = anxiety. Seems legit. With that idea, you could spend years trying to heal anxiety from the logical angle of *fear of being alone caused it*. But in reality, you could be following the wrong lead. Emotions are not logical. That's why it often takes a totally different approach—muscle testing—to get to the real root of what's going on.

So many times I've worked with clients who have been going to therapy for ten or twenty years to work through something like repressed emotions from their parents' divorce, only to find out later, through tapping into their subconscious mind, that their anxiety was linked to something completely different, like the birth of a sibling (which they don't even recall being traumatic). The clues and information we discover in the subconscious can be surprising, and my clients usually doubt or question it at first. But then, when they clear the energy connected to that information, they see great improvement.

While the brain will always aim to untangle a challenge in the most logical way, I find that there is often no logical reason for what actually causes anxiety and what doesn't, and why it occurs in some people and not others. I often see certain patterns that do make sense, such as certain ages and experiences coming up where I can say, "Yes, of course that would cause anxiety!" However, by using the technique of muscle testing, I just as often help my clients identify ages and experiences where there is no conscious connection to the anxiety, but clearing the emotional energy connected to it helps them. I'll show you what I mean in the following example.

When Jack came to me for help with panic attacks, he told me that ever since he'd had a bad experience at the doctor's office when he was eight, he'd been fearful all the time. After that visit, he developed some OCD-type symptoms and was afraid to touch things in case he might get sick and have to go back to the doctor. That seemed to make total sense. However, he had been to therapy and had even done hypnosis for that experience for years, but he saw no improvement in the panic attacks. As we worked with muscle testing, just like you'll be learning to do shortly, we learned that his panic attacks were actually tied to a few different ages in his life. This is quite common. There is rarely one reason for or cause of anxiety. It's more like a web of energies that needs to be cleared.

The other ages we identified through muscle testing were two and four years old. Jack didn't remember anything traumatic from those times, but when I started asking questions, he realized that he'd had a sibling born at each of those ages. Now, to the adult brain that might seem like a happy time! And when Jack asked his mom how he'd reacted, she said that he'd loved meeting his new siblings. But what Jack and I figured out was that during those two times, there had been a lot of emphasis put on hand washing to protect the new siblings. It really scared Jack that everyone in the house was so afraid of illness, and it impacted him greatly. Perhaps those were the original sources of the panic that got retriggered later when he had the negative experience at the doctor's office at age eight. The original experience (or experiences) might seem small in the big picture of life, but the age at which we had the experience and the ability we possessed at the time to process life's difficulties can strongly influence how greatly we are affected by it.

When I started working with Jack to release stuck emotions (chapter 6), clear unprocessed experiences from his past (chapter 7), and change harmful beliefs (chapter 8) related to experiences around these ages, he saw an immediate shift. You will be learning how to do this too.

Use the Subconscious Mind to Release Anxiety

We've already acknowledged how great it is that our subconscious mind often does things without us needing to think about them. However, a problem arises when the rules in your subconscious mind (which were created as a child) clash strongly with what your (adult-programmed) conscious mind is trying to achieve—overcoming anxiety.

The subconscious mind will direct your behavior according to its programming and rules and adhere to them no matter what. That's how the subconscious "protects" us or does what it believes is good for us. If, for some reason, the subconscious mind believes it's *better* to have anxiety than to release it, it will stick to that rule and direct your behavior in accordance with it. This type of message can prevent you from being totally aligned with your goal of healing.

My client Alyssa struggled with this exact predicament. For her, anxiety began in high school. Even though she first noticed it at age sixteen, she said it seemed to come on for no apparent reason. What we discovered for Alyssa was that anxiety was sometimes the only way she felt that she could tell her friends no. Alyssa was such a people-pleaser that saying no to others was nearly impossible for her, but her friends were so compassionate and understanding about the anxiety that she felt a sense of relief. She could easily say she didn't want to attend a party or help a friend with their homework due to anxiety, and no one would question it. In addition, her parents no longer put any pressure on her about grades, as they were just happy that she could make it to school.

We discovered that there was some programming in her subconscious mind that was giving her the message that anxiety was the only way she could say no to others. Of course, there were in fact other ways that she could have said no, but to her subconscious mind, having anxiety was the best way to avoid doing so! That became her body's steadfast belief, and her subconscious helped create anxiety in order to fulfill it. If she started to have a hard time saying no, the anxiety would begin to come on strongly.

This pattern was hidden in her subconscious until we brought it to light. In order to change the rules we live by and react from, we need to actually *identify* the programming first. This is what we did for Alyssa, and it almost instantly decreased her anxiety dramatically. You will learn more about how to do this throughout the entire book.

During my own healing, the information I found in my subconscious was mind-blowing and sometimes embarrassing. But through working with it, I discovered energies to release that I would not have likely found using my conscious thought process. This allowed me to work on issues I'd never been aware of, and in turn, to see results I'd never gotten before.

Learning to communicate with your subconscious mind is a wild ride, but it's worth every twisty turn. Keep an open and curious mind and you'll see just what I mean.

Use Muscle Testing to Access Your Subconscious Mind

Throughout the healing process in this book, I will help you use the simple technique of muscle testing to tap into your subconscious mind. This will help you identify and release emotional blockages that you've likely never addressed before and get results you haven't in the past. Muscle testing will essentially tell you exactly what you need to do for your healing. How cool is that?

Muscle testing is an energy detection technique, not an energy healing technique. We use it to detect or identify *what* to clear, and then use the energy therapy techniques you'll be learning to actually clear them. Muscle testing and energy therapy techniques work together, just like the conscious and subconscious minds do. You can heal by working with just one or the other technique, but when you combine both, you have a powerful team behind you. Muscle testing will give you so many clues as to which stuck emotions, unprocessed experiences, and harmful beliefs to clear (all of which we'll be covering thoroughly in chapters 6–8).

Now that I've been using muscle testing for a long time, I see it as training wheels for the intuition. I get so much of my information naturally and intuitively now, but muscle testing was the first way I learned to tap into the hidden wisdom I already had.

Let's talk about what muscle testing is and how it works, and then, most importantly, how to use it in order to release anxiety.

As you've learned, the body itself is made up of pure energy. Our entire system is essentially a type of electrical system. This system influences the energetic interaction between our physical body and our subconscious mind. I like to think of the nervous system as a long antenna picking up on energetic frequencies in our environment—energies that are too subtle even for scientific instruments to measure. That electrical (or energy) system, which is connected to our subconscious mind, responds and reacts to all other energies, positive and negative. If something impacts our electrical system in a way that does not help maintain or enhance our body's energetic balance (in other words, it's not positive for or congruent with our body), then our body's energy system will temporarily "short-circuit," affecting the electrical (or energetic) flow running through our muscles, glands, and other organs (just like we learned in chapter 1). Some of the things that can affect our electrical system are thoughts, emotions, foods, and other substances.

In order to find out what our subconscious mind and body are in agreement or resonance with, we can ask it questions directly. After asking the questions, we'll use our body's muscles' responses to determine what our body's answers are (hence the term "muscle testing"). Muscle testing is simply a super cool way to ask our body questions and get clear answers that we couldn't decipher on our own. It's like having a direct phone line to our subconscious mind.

Here is how muscle testing works:

- If we make a statement that our body and subconscious mind *agrees with* at a core level (meaning the statement is true for us), our electrical system will continue flowing without a hitch and our muscles will retain their full strength.

- If we make a statement that our body and subconscious mind *disagrees with* at a core level (meaning the statement is not true for us), our energy system will temporarily short-circuit and our muscles will quickly weaken or lock up. This temporary state is not dangerous at all.

Each of these reactions gives us a way to interpret what our body is saying to us.

Very Important Note: There is no reason to panic if muscle testing isn't an instant success for you. While many people take to it quite easily, it took me almost a year to master it. Throughout the book, I give you many ways to continue your healing journey without using muscle testing. This is simply a helpful tool to guide you along, but is not necessary in order to have success with my approach.

Two Ways to Muscle-Test

There are endless muscle-testing techniques out there, but I typically teach the following two ways, which I find to be the easiest for most people to learn. Try to be curious and relaxed as you practice. Don't worry about doing it perfectly. We are using this tool because it's far better than guessing, like you've been doing up until now; but our lives don't depend on its accuracy, so don't put a ton of pressure on yourself during the process.

The Standing Test

One way of muscle testing that is typically easy for beginners to learn is called the *Standing Test*. It works on the following basis. Your thoughts and emotions produce a certain response in your nervous system, affecting your motor response (movement of your body). The unconscious part of you, which isn't using logic or rational thought, will naturally be drawn to something that it sees as positive or the truth and will naturally be repelled by something that it doesn't read as truthful for you.

If you ask questions when your body is in a relaxed but standing position (but is still able to move without obstruction), it will involuntarily sway—either slightly backward or slightly forward—which will help you determine if it is aligned with something or not. Remember, words are just energy, so using them will create some kind of response in the body.

The Standing Test can also be done in a chair if you aren't mobile. With this technique we are essentially using your body as a pendulum.

1. Stand or sit up straight, with your feet about shoulder-width apart and pointing directly forward. Ensure that both feet are directly forward and neither is slightly

turned in or out. Relax your body, with your hands down at your sides. Close your eyes if you are able to stand safely with your eyes closed. Take a big, deep breath.

2. Now you are ready to ask your body some questions. Your energy system will be picking up on the energy of what you are saying and reacting to the questions involuntarily.

First, you're going to make sure you get an accurate base test. This is just to make sure your body is responding properly so you can trust the rest of the testing and know it's accurate.

Say this statement out loud: *Show me a yes.* Your body should involuntarily tip slightly forward, meaning "yes." It is showing you that it's in alignment or resonance with what you are saying. Think of this as a head nod for "yes," but with your whole body. Next, say this statement out loud: *Show me a no.* Your body should involuntarily tip slightly backward, meaning "no." It is showing you that it is rejecting or is repelled by what you're saying.

You might experience some personal variations to the standard forward or backward responses. For example, I have a few clients who kind of swing and lean to the left for "yes" and stay pretty neutral for "no." We figured out that this was just their body's own unique response, and we embraced it. We get accurate answers now that we know exactly how their body gives us a yes or a no. Be open to your own variations too.

If you are getting the total opposite responses to what you should (meaning backward for "yes" and forward for "no"), it is most likely because your energy is scrambled and is not balanced enough. Take a few deep breaths, and relax. It can be helpful to tap your thymus gland for thirty seconds to a minute. Being too cerebral interferes with the process of letting your body respond naturally. Just keep trying. It can take some time to trust this process and let it happen, especially if you like to be in control. Again, it took a long time and a lot of practice for me to get good at it.

3. Let's play around with this technique just a little bit more so you can see how helpful it can be.

Say this statement out loud and notice your body's response: *It's safe for me to heal from anxiety.* Alternatively, you can ask it in question form and notice your body's response. The format you use to get a response doesn't matter at all, so choose whatever feels more natural to you—either a question or a statement.

Just relax and allow your body to naturally sway either forward or backward gently. This is how it will give you your answer. This will happen without you consciously doing anything, so if you analyze it or try to "help," it will interfere with the process. If your body leans forward slightly, your subconscious mind and body are essentially saying, "Yes, I'm in agreement with what you just said." This means that at a core level your body believes it's safe for you to heal and that you agree with the statement at a deep, subconscious level. Yay! That's what we want, although this response is pretty rare.

If your body tips or pulls backward, moving away from the statement, then your subconscious mind and body are saying, "No, it's not safe for me to heal." Don't worry though. This is not a fact; it's only a belief. And it's actually the most common response I see with clients. This is only what your body is currently in agreement with, which can be changed. That's why we're here doing this work. If that's your answer, you might be surprised to find out that it is the norm. In order to heal, we'll need your body and your subconscious mind to agree at a core level that it's safe to heal so you can move forward without resistance. The good news is that you'll be learning how to clear this belief (along with lots of other beliefs that might be blocking you) later in chapter 8. I'll be sharing common beliefs that need to be changed based on the thousands of client sessions I've conducted. I'll also show you how to discover some for yourself.

When muscle testing, it's super important to relax, detach from the possible answer, and focus only on the question or statement. Because your body responds to the energy of thoughts, emotions, and more, if you are thinking about a bunch of things, including what the answer will be, it will influence the answer. I totally get that human beings love to analyze, but for this tool to be of use to you, try to really let go and stay open.

The O-Ring Test

I'm going to share one more muscle-testing method with you as an alternative to the Standing Test. I call this the *O-Ring Test*. With your dominant hand, touch the pad of your thumb to the pad of your middle finger to create an "O" shape. Don't press too firmly. Now insert the pointer finger from your other hand so it's resting where the thumb and middle finger join. It will look a little like your pointer finger is a fishing hook. Using medium pressure, pull away from the O-ring with your pointer finger to try to break the seal of your "O."

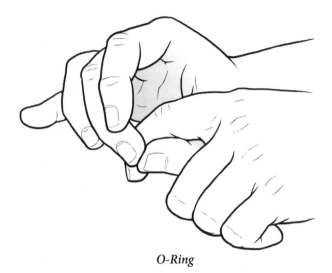

O-Ring

Exactly as you did with the Standing Test, you're going to either formulate yes-no statements or ask your body yes-no questions. After you make a statement or ask a question, you'll use the pointer finger "hook" to try to pull the O-ring open. When you pull with your "hook" finger after verbalizing the question or statement, gauge your body's response to determine what answer your subconscious is giving you. You don't want to use excessive force to do this, as surely you could break the seal of your "O" if you tried hard enough. Rather, you want to tug away from your hand and see if the "o" gives way fairly easily. You are essentially trying to see if the muscles in the O-ring hand weaken.

When you did the Standing Test, tipping forward was your body's "yes" response and tipping backward was your body's "no." With the O-Ring Test, your body is saying "yes" or "I'm in agreement with the question or statement" when your "O" formation stays strong without any difficulty. This means that you don't feel any "give" in the O-ring. If your "O" feels like it loses some strength and wants to open or break apart under the pressure, your muscle is temporarily short-circuiting (like we talked about at the beginning of this chapter). Your body is saying "no" or "I'm not in agreement with the question or statement."

Muscle testing with the O-ring is not a fight between your fingers. You are simply noticing if the "O" weakens with slight pressure from your "hook" finger. It may take some time to get the right calibration, like getting the flame on a gas stove just right. With practice, you'll find the balance that works right for you.

To make things easy, here is a quick key to figuring out what your body is communicating through muscle testing:

Standing Test:
Forward = "Yes, I agree."
Backward = "No, I don't agree."

O-Ring Test:
"O" stays strong under pressure = "Yes, I agree."
"O" breaks under pressure = "No, I don't agree."

There are tons of muscle-testing techniques available out there. While the Standing Test and the O-Ring Test are two of my favorites, you could explore muscle testing much further on your own if you have the interest. You can also try pendulum testing, an alternative to muscle testing that may be easier for you. I'll share that next.

I can't stress enough the value of this tool, but I also don't want to imply that everyone learns it easily right away. In fact, I first learned muscle testing in a class where I was the only one out of about thirty people who couldn't seem to master it. I almost gave up on it out of frustration, but I kept trying, and over time it just kind of clicked. Whether you master muscle testing instantly or not, you can still move forward with the approach outlined in the following chapters.

An Alternative to Muscle Testing: Pendulum Testing

I'm going to quickly share an alternative method to tap into the subconscious mind. It's the equivalent of muscle testing, but some people find it easier to do. This technique is called *pendulum testing*. Instead of using your body for this testing, you will be using a pendulum, which will act as a conduit for your own energy. To start, you will need a necklace chain or a string with a weighted object looped through it. You can use a necklace with a pendant, or if you don't have that, just loop a piece of string through a bolt. It needs to be long enough to hang down and swing freely, but there are no requirements for length or weight. Now, using a few fingers, simply hold your chain or string with the pendulum out in front of you and allow it to dangle down. The string or chain should be hanging down from your fingertips, with the weighted object at the bottom.

Exactly as you did with the Standing Test and the O-Ring Test, you're going to either formulate yes-no statements or ask your pendulum yes-no questions. Instead of your body swaying, as it did with the Standing Test, it will be your pendulum that sways in response to your energy. It is helpful to first "program" your pendulum by establishing what it will do for a "yes" response and what it will do for a "no" response. You can do this by saying, "Show me a yes" and then watching what your pendulum does. Then say, "Show me a no" and observe that as well. The pendulum will typically sway forward away from your body and then back toward your body for a "yes" and sway from side to side horizontally for a "no." However, your "yes" and "no" responses may be different. For instance, your pendulum may make circles for a "yes" and remain still for a "no." Any response is fine as long as you can determine what the pendulum does for each response.

After you make the statement or ask the question, watch to see what the pendulum does. Make sure your arm is somewhat relaxed (you can rest an elbow on the table), and allow the pendulum to swing naturally. Gauge the pendulum's response to figure out what answer your subconscious is relaying to you.

With pendulum testing, your body is saying "yes" or "I'm in resonance" with the question when the pendulum is exhibiting whatever your "yes" response is. If your pendulum does whatever your "no" response is, then your energy is temporarily short-circuiting, like we talked about at the beginning of this chapter. Your body is saying "no" or "I'm not in resonance" with the question or statement.

Throughout this book, I'm going to use the term *muscle testing* only to keep things simple, but please know that muscle testing and pendulum testing are completely interchangeable, so feel free to use the latter if it works better for you.

Tips for Muscle Testing

Because I had such a difficult time at first with muscle testing, I discovered many tricks to make the technique as accurate as possible. But remember, this is just a useful tool. The best thing you can do is relax while using it. Here are some tips for you:

- Make sure you're well hydrated. Electricity requires water, and if you're dehydrated, your energy system won't be working the way it should, making it difficult to get clear answers.

- Ask the question in a different way if you aren't getting a clear answer. Sometimes the body won't respond if we're not on the right track or our question needs to be tweaked slightly. Just change the way you ask the question, similarly to how you would reword something slightly if you explained it to a friend and they were confused.

- Make sure to take a deep breath and pause in between questions to allow your body and brain to recalibrate. Going too fast will lead to sensory overload and your system will freeze up, yielding confusing answers.

- Move away from electronics, as they can interfere with your body's energetic flow.

- Make statements or ask questions using only affirmative language. For example, if you are trying to find out if you believe deep down that you *can* heal, use the statement *I can heal* and see how your body responds, instead of using *I can't heal.* It is confusing to the body to use negatives in this way while muscle testing.

- Caution: Do not use the muscle-testing technique to try to predict the future, win the lottery, confirm for yourself if you were abused or neglected as a child, or make major life decisions. The answers won't be accurate, and making decisions based on muscle testing can be dangerous—I and many other very proficient muscle testers can tell you that from experience! Muscle testing should be used as a tool only to see what your body is in *resonance* with, so you can change and release emotional energies that are no longer serving you.

- We'll be using muscle testing throughout the coming chapters, so you'll have lots of opportunities to practice the technique. Just be patient and open until you get the hang of it. Until then, I'll still be showing you how to identify energy blockages and clear them even without muscle testing. You don't need muscle testing to heal, but if you can get the hang of it, I know you'll find it very useful.

Now that you understand the basics of emotions and the energy system and the art of muscle testing, you are ready to officially begin the adventure of healing. Let's start with calming and retraining your body. Follow me.

Summary

While anxiety can be a very confusing and complex issue, your body actually has so much information and wisdom about what's causing or contributing to it. The subconscious mind may have programming that is making it difficult for you to overcome anxiety and heal.

The good news is that by tapping into your subconscious mind, you can have great success and even expedite your healing. Muscle testing and pendulum testing are two great tools to help you do that.

Section II

* * * * * * * * * * * * * * *

Start Healing Now

Chapter Four

* * * * * * * * * * * * * *

Calm and Retrain Your Body

In this chapter, we're going to delve further into the body's fight, flight, or freeze response (which I call the freak-out response) to help you understand why it has been so darn hard for you to heal. What most people describe as overwhelm is actually part of this dynamic, which causes people to feel stuck in a frozen state, unable to help themselves. This dynamic can create a perpetual cycle of self-sabotage.

We'll be focusing on a specific protocol for calming the freak-out response in your body, which essentially acts as a retraining program. I'm going to teach you some very easy-to-implement techniques, as well as suggest a simple way to use them as a daily program. In this chapter, you'll take your very first step toward healing.

The Fight, Flight, or Freeze Response

The fight, flight or freeze response (aka the freak-out response) is governed by the part of the energy system called the triple warmer meridian. To help you understand the triple warmer meridian better, think of it as an inner protective "papa bear." When you hold unresolved emotional experiences in your body, you can become suspended in a place where the triple warmer meridian is in a state of panic or overdrive, trying to protect you from having those things happen again, whether or not that's even a consideration. When the triple warmer is hard at work protecting you, you are in freak-out mode. This is essentially a state of stress, which is orchestrated by the sympathetic nervous system.

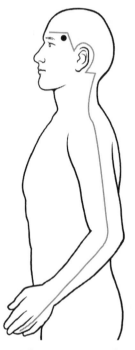

Triple Warmer Meridian

There are three kinds of involuntary responses people typically have when they are scared: fight (you get pumped up and want to fight the current situation), flight (you want to run away as fast as you can), or freeze (you become frozen and can't do anything at all). Some of us tend toward one response more than the others or embody all three at different times depending on the situation. I am an escape artist at heart. Give me a problem, a difficult emotion, or anything that overwhelms me and my first instinct will always be to book a vacation. If I can't do that, I'll want to go out to dinner. Those are examples of "flight." Can't leave the house? In that case, I'd lean toward wanting to do nothing at all to help myself. I'd take a bath. Dawdle around. Ignore what's going on. Those are examples of "freeze." If I acted on these tendencies, it would not be a healthy pattern at all.

It's important to realize that stress can sometimes be beneficial. This is the case when we are in true danger and need a surge of chemicals to help us fight (defend ourselves), take flight (escape the situation), or freeze (blend in or hide) to avoid the danger and stay safe.

A great example of how the fight, flight, or freeze response *should* work can be observed in animals in the wild. When animals are in danger, they go into fight, flight, or freeze mode as a way to escape that danger (tigers "fight," rabbits "freeze," and antelope take "flight"). But when the dangerous situation is over, they shake or tremble to discharge the stress. Humans, however, aren't quite as good at the stress-releasing process. Because of how we've evolved in our fast-paced culture, our system gets to a point where it can't determine the difference between stresses from an actual danger or threat and those stemming from unresolved emotional baggage. To the body, it's all just "stressful." In addition, we typically don't learn stress-relief techniques early on, so we often end up with no way to release the stress and move forward. This causes us to get stuck in freak-out mode, which not only can create anxiety but can prevent us from healing from it too.

Are you starting to have more compassion for yourself about why you've been stuck? I seriously hope so!

How Fight, Flight, or Freeze Affects You Physically

While some people may believe that anxiety is "all in your head," I'm going to illustrate why that couldn't be further from the truth.

Remember, storing old emotional energy in the body can cause the body to get suspended in fight, flight, or freeze mode. During the fight, flight, or freeze response, the triple warmer meridian is doing everything it can to protect us (like a papa bear does for his cub), but in doing so, the sympathetic nervous system goes into stress mode. This is the total opposite of healing mode.

The fight, flight, or freeze response triggers the following physiological stress reactions:

- Blood is shunted away from the gastrointestinal tract, spleen, and other nonvital organs.

- The body produces additional glucose.

- The immune system becomes suppressed, in part through the production of high cortisol levels brought on by the release of adrenaline.

- The areas of the brain related to short- and long-term memory are affected.

- Heart rate and blood pressure increase.

If we don't resolve the emotional baggage that contributed to creating this dynamic, we may get stuck in this perpetual state, which is exactly what happens in the case of anxiety. As a reminder, emotions or stress are not problems in and of themselves. They are totally normal. The challenge comes in how our body's energy system *reacts* to those stressful influences, because that causes imbalances that can create anxiety.

The body has an amazing ability to protect and defend itself (via the fight, flight, or freeze response) and also to heal and repair itself. The tricky thing is that these processes cannot happen simultaneously. The body can settle into full healing mode only once we take it out of crisis, or freak-out, mode. But before you start to worry, let me reassure you that this doesn't in any way mean that you have to be totally calm or void of all stress in order to heal. It simply means that it is your job to do the reprogramming necessary to make your body feel as safe and relaxed as possible. That's what we're going to begin walking through together now.

Calm and Retrain Your Body

The most effective way to begin healing anxiety is by turning off the fight, flight, or freeze response. In other words, you need to convince the triple warmer meridian that it's safe to move from freak-out mode to chill-out mode so you can relax and live your life.

As you work to turn off the fight, flight, or freeze response, you are actually initiating a relaxed state in your system. When you are relaxed, your parasympathetic nervous system is utilizing its "rest and digest" function. You are in healing mode. Your nervous system is absolutely key to this process.

There are ways we can help ourselves get to a calm and relaxed state:

Step 1: Calm and Retrain Your Body's Freak-Out Response

Using specific exercises that you'll learn in this chapter, you can retrain your triple warmer meridian to calm down and help elicit the relaxation response instead of the freak-out response.

Step 2: Address the Root of Anxiety

In section 3, we'll be clearing old emotional energies that helped create anxiety in the first place. All emotional baggage can disrupt your energy system and trigger the fight, flight, or freeze response in your body. This is why it's essential to work with both steps that I've described.

We are going to start with the calming and retraining. If we can get your body to shift even a little bit in the direction of relaxation, it will be so much easier to clear the emotional baggage that has been stored in your body for a long time.

The relaxation response can be achieved in many ways, including meditation, yoga, qi gong, and more. However, during my own healing journey I found it nearly impossible to do any of those things. I was actually *too* unrelaxed to be relaxed!

My own process is effective because it doesn't require any great amount of concentration or discipline—and it doesn't require you to sit still. It helps you begin to shift the *energy* of fight, flight, or freeze so you can more easily do the deeper work of going back to clear the emotional energies that caused the response in the first place.

Once you do these steps of calming and retraining your body and also release the emotional energies that created anxiety (chapters 6–8), you will no longer have to be afraid of life. You will no longer need to cope with triggers because you will have changed your body's entire relationship to them and the world around you. Anxiety relief is on its way!

A Daily Program: Calm and Retrain Your Body

The most important thing about calming the freak-out response is that it must be done with consistency. The body's freak-out mode should be thought of as a bad habit that can be broken only with gentle but persistent dedication. I liken this retraining process to potty-training a puppy. If you've ever done it, you know it's all about consistency, persistence, and more consistency. Oh yes, and patience! When a puppy goes to the bathroom in the wrong place, you have to show them the right thing to do—over and over. You can't decide to do it only sometimes, or the training won't work. Your energy system is exactly the same. Imagine you are the puppy. When your body is in freak-out mode, you need to show it a better alternative (relaxation mode) over and over again until that becomes the default response. By using these simple techniques throughout each day, you'll be saying to your body, *Hey, let's do this calming thing now instead of that freaking-out thing we've been doing.*

Triple warmer energy is resistant to change and highly sensitive to overwhelm, so take tiny, gentle steps. It's the most effective way of coaxing the triple warmer meridian to cooperate with your attempt to change your body's long-held freak-out pattern. While consistency is a must, that certainly doesn't mean you have to use the following techniques for hours at a time. It's actually more effective to use them for short amounts of time multiple times each day. This is all about setting a new and healthier habit, which is going to require some training.

The Techniques

You'll be using the following three techniques throughout each day to begin calming and retraining your body. Each technique is super simple and takes only a couple minutes to perform. Play around with all of them and see which ones work best for you. You'll know you've found an effective technique when you feel your energy shift, your body calms down, and your thinking becomes clearer.

(1) Forehead Rest

When we go into freak-out mode, a large amount of blood leaves the frontal lobes of the brain, which clouds our thinking and makes it difficult to talk ourselves into calming down. But you already know this if you've ever tried to use logic to get yourself out of a panic. I learned this exercise from Donna Eden.[3] It uses the electromagnetic energy in your fingertips to help draw the blood back up to your frontal lobes so you can calm down and think of what to do for yourself next.

Rest your fingertips very gently on your forehead area above the eyebrows. I like to rest my thumbs on my temples (because the temples are connected to the triple warmer meridian) and cup my palms over my eyes. This pose will look like you're playing peekaboo with a baby. Just hold your hands this way and breathe for thirty seconds to a few minutes, or until you feel a slight "pulsing" in your fingertips or until you feel calmer.

(2) Triple Warmer Meridian Trace

When the triple warmer meridian becomes overcharged, your body is likely to feel full of adrenaline and panic. Luckily, there is a great way to tame this meridian and get it to calm down. We can do this by tracing backward over the pathway of the triple warmer meridian. This will gently release or draw out any excess energy that is not needed in the moment.

Place your hands against either side of your face so your fingertips are resting on your temples and your palms are resting on your cheeks. Now slowly and deliberately trace with your hands up and around your ears (staying in contact with your head) and then pull them down the sides of your neck until you reach your shoulders. Now lift your hands off and cross your arms so each hand is resting on the opposite shoulder, then slide each hand down an arm in a self-hug position, end-

---

3. Donna Eden, with David Feinstein, *Energy Medicine: How to Use Your Body's Energies for Optimum Health and Vitality* (London: Piatkus, 1999).

ing when you are holding your own hands in any way that feels natural to you. Repeat the entire motion several more times.

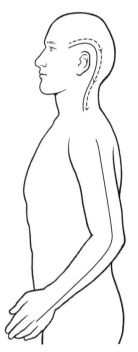

Triple Warmer Meridian Trace

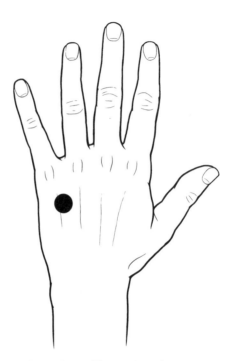

Panic Point (Gamut Point)

(3) Use the Panic Point

There is a magic place on the top of either hand that is very helpful for calming the body down. It's about halfway down the top of the hand in between the pinky and ring fingers, and is located right along the triple warmer meridian line. By tapping or rubbing this spot, called the *gamut point*, we can actually calm down its energy, which will have a direct effect on the body. Simply tap or rub this spot using three or four fingers of your other hand. Use this technique along with deep breaths. This one is perfect to do under a restaurant table or a desk. Because this spot is located directly on the energy pathway of the triple warmer meridian, working with it actually sends a message to that energy force to back off from being in overprotective mode and chill out.

When and For How Long to Use the Techniques

In an effort to change the habits and patterns of the triple warmer meridian, exercises should be done at least three times a day, preferably in the morning, at midday, and in the evening. But I don't have any strict rules, so do whatever works for you in terms of timing.

You already know the great foundational practices from chapter 1 (grounding, eye trace, and thymus tapping), which will help balance your energy and give you a sturdy healing foundation to work with. Hopefully you've gotten into a habit of doing those daily. Now we're going to be adding the specific calming and retraining techniques you just learned into your daily routine.

There are a couple ways you'll integrate the three new techniques you just learned.

First: Anytime you get triggered into panic or stress mode, you must immediately practice a calming technique: the forehead rest, triple warmer meridian trace, or panic point. It doesn't matter which one, so choose whatever you're called to use. This is the only way you can show your body what to do instead of panicking. Eventually, if this is done consistently (at least thirty days in a row), you will start to feel a shift in your body's response to stress.

Second: You will set a timer or make a mental note to integrate the techniques into your day at three different time intervals, such as in the morning (when you wake up), at noon, and in the evening (before bed). The times definitely don't have to be exact, but try to space them as evenly as you can. Essentially, you'll choose a technique at each time of day and practice it for at least two minutes each time (a total of six minutes a day). Aim to increase your time to a total of fifteen minutes a day (five minutes for each exercise).

Using the techniques both on an as-needed basis and also consistently three times a day is going to do wonders for re-training your system to be calm. It's a gentle reminder to do "this" (be calm) instead of "that" (freak-out mode). And just like potty-training a puppy, it'll pay off if you stick with it! Before you know it, your body will be relaxing on its own.

Summary

It is essential to address the body's fight, flight, or freeze response (aka the freak-out response) in order to completely release anxiety from the body. During times of stress or trauma, it is totally normal for the body to go into fight, flight, or freeze mode. However, when the body remains suspended in that state, it can make it difficult to heal from anxiety or can contribute to it. To be successful in clearing anxiety, we must begin by working with the triple warmer energy (responsible for the fight, flight, or freeze response). Calming this response is a key to our anxiety-healing protocol. This is essentially a retraining program for the body.

Next, you'll learn how to deal with your present feelings in a whole new way. Then you'll be ready to release deep-seated emotional blockages for full and complete healing. You're getting there!

* * * * * * * * * * * * * * * *

Chapter Five

Deal With Your Feelings

Emotions are a natural part of being human. Although I used to resist dealing with my feelings because it was so uncomfortable for me, I now understand the cost of doing so: anxiety, and sometimes even physical illness. Suppressing emotions like anger, fear, and sadness is just too much for our bodies to bear. In order to come fully into our wellbeing we must have tools to deal with our emotions in the present moment. Even if you've never done this before, it's not too late to start. In fact, dealing with your feelings is the first step in teaching your body to *let go* of them instead of *hold on* to them. Just this one piece— dealing with your emotions so they don't get suppressed and manifest as anxiety—can have a huge and positive impact on your life—and quickly!

Since the best place to start is always right where you are, you'll learn in this chapter exactly what to do with your difficult emotions—essentially, anxiety—so you can start feeling better right away. I'm going to teach you two powerful techniques for dealing with your feelings in the present moment: Emotional Freedom Technique (EFT) and Chakra Tapping, which can be used interchangeably.

Then, in the next chapter, you'll learn how to go back into your past and do even deeper work to release emotions you've been carrying for a long time—maybe even your whole life. But don't worry, that process is going to be a lot easier than you think!

Emotions: The Basics

When we go through experiences in life, we are really just *feeling* our way through them. When we have upsetting experiences, we might feel sad, angry, or frustrated. Those are all emotions that we might think of as "negative" or "bad," but emotions are harmless in and of themselves—as long as they keep flowing and don't get stuck. In fact, emotions are meant to be fluid, not frozen. The word *emotion* itself comes from the Latin *emovēre*, "to disturb," which is from the Latin *e-* + *movēre*, "to move." But when emotions are suppressed instead of dealt with as they come up, the experience of prolonged feelings can create anxiety.

You've already learned that when an animal in the wild experiences a stressful event, they shake, tremble, run, or do other physical activities to discharge the effect of the stress chemicals on their body. Our human tendency is to do this too, but we are often encouraged to "calm down," "get it together," "stop being so sensitive," "grow up," and "suck it up." It may be that you were told these things as a child or that you're naturally uncomfortable with feeling your feelings and have been telling yourself these things all along. Either way, if we don't feel, process, and release the strong emotions we feel, they can stay frozen in our system, getting triggered and retriggered throughout our lives. Some of the emotions we felt during difficult and stressful times could remain active and vibrating inside of us.

In order to completely change our body's pattern of creating anxiety, we need to start dealing with our emotions right now. You'll want to use the following techniques whenever you are experiencing difficult emotions—from feeling anxious for "no reason" to being angry because someone did something to hurt you. I remind my clients all the time that "if you are sitting around feeling yucky, you might as well use the techniques to help it move out while you're sitting there!" The idea behind this is to actually move the energy that's coming up out of your body. This may be a new concept to you, but dealing with your feelings as they come up is going to make all the difference for healing anxiety.

Emotional Freedom Technique (EFT)— The Easy Amy Way!

EFT is one of my very favorite ways to deal with emotions because it's easy to use, you don't need anything but yourself to do it, and it's effective. There are so many applications for EFT that I pretty much use it for everything! When I first learned EFT, I found it complicated and strange. I didn't resonate with it at all. A practitioner I was working with performed EFT on me to help release some fear I was having, and I just sat there confused. While I did feel better afterward, I left her office that day and never thought about it again. She didn't explain to me that I could use it for myself, on myself, or that it could actually be simple! Many years later when I rediscovered the technique, I learned to keep it simple and use it on my own, and now I use it almost every day. What I'm going to do now is teach you the basic way to use it to address all the feelings you may be struggling with *right now*. Then, in the next chapter, you'll learn how to build on this basic form and go deeper to release emotions from your past as well.

EFT gives us an opportunity to focus on the feelings that are coming up in the moment instead of ignoring and suppressing them. Using EFT, we go through the healthy process of dealing with and letting go of our emotions. This is done very gently. As we work with our emotions using EFT, we are likely to have conscious realizations, cognitive shifts, and perspective changes about our feelings during the process. This often helps us to feel better, not only because we are releasing the suppressed emotions, but also because we become less stressed and panicked about our overall situation. Many times, new clients tell me they are worried about feeling their feelings because they fear they'll be opening Pandora's box. But the truth is that you've already been feeling the feelings (hence the anxiety), so the only thing you are doing now is really dealing with them and clearing them.

What Is EFT?

EFT is a simple and effective tool based on the meridian system, a system of energy pathways in the body originating in Chinese medicine thousands of years ago. It combines the principles of acupuncture (without the needles) and talking! EFT was founded in the early 1990s by Stanford graduate and engineer Gary Craig.[4] The technique is based on Thought Field Therapy, which Craig learned from Dr. Roger Callahan. Callahan's specific process of tapping sequentially on acupuncture points while recalling fearful memories was groundbreaking but too complicated for people to use on their own. Gary Craig was able to simplify the process and make it accessible to everyone in the form of EFT. It's one of the simplest and most effective tools I've ever utilized!

Meridians in the body are energy pathways that are woven together to form a larger network. Along the meridians, there are special points commonly used in acupuncture that can be

---

4. Gary Craig, "What Is EFT? Theory, Science, and Uses," Official EFT, https://www.emofree.com/eft-tutorial/tapping-basics/what-is-eft.html.

accessed to move energy and remove blockages. Where there is an energetic imbalance, there is a corresponding blockage in the meridian system, which contributes to emotional and physical symptoms. Gently tapping on these points with the fingertips works to release the blockages and restore balance.

Gary Craig states that the cause of all negative emotion is an imbalance in the energy system. Let me share more about what that means by giving you an example. Imagine that two people have the same experience—for example, being teased in school about their clothes—and one is greatly affected by it (left with feelings of sadness or worthlessness) while the other one isn't. This is due to the equivalent of a metaphorical *bzzzt* (think little electrical zap) that happens in the energy system at the time of the emotional stress. This phenomenon, and whether it occurs in any given situation, is unique to each person's individual system. It's not exactly what happens to us or the emotions we feel that cause a problem for us. It's more the way our energy system reacts to a specific emotional experience or trauma. If we get that disturbance, or *bzzzt*, in our energy system, the experience and emotions are more likely to get stuck and affect us negatively. Some of us simply have a greater tendency for our energy flow to get disrupted or imbalanced during such experiences.

EFT gives us a way to remedy the metaphorical *bzzzt* in the energy system that imbalanced things in the first place. The even better news is that the more your energy system becomes balanced through this work, the less likely it is that you'll be affected in the same way by experiences in the future.

By restoring balance to our body's energy system in relationship to our emotions, we are addressing and releasing the imbalanced energies that are directly contributing to anxiety.

This is my favorite analogy to explain how EFT works. Imagine your dog, Rufus, totally freaks out every time the mailman comes to the door. Each day you tell Rufus in your most calming voice that he's okay and safe around Mr. Mailman, but chances are Rufus will just look at you like you don't know what you're talking about and continue to bark in fear. But if you kneel down next to him and pat him, calming him at the same time he is looking at this scary, mean mailman, you'll be sending a strong signal to his body that he is safe and okay even while facing this "danger" (Mr. Mailman and his mean mailbag). You are changing how Rufus feels about this thing that is usually stressful, and ultimately you are changing the pattern of what happens to Rufus in his body when he sees the mailman. His system is now reprogramming itself to be okay and balanced in the presence of Mr. Mailman. You are not changing the circumstance but rather the reaction in the body. We're basically doing the same thing for you. We're changing what happens to you in your energy body when you are feeling difficult emotions.

I have often had new clients tell me they tried EFT before but didn't like it. I always end up getting them hooked on the "Easy Amy Way"! I teach EFT to kids as young as five years old, so anyone can learn it easily. The key is to keep the process simple. This is not a technique with strict rules, so have fun! If you do, you'll have a powerful tool that you can use any time, anywhere.

Where to Tap: The Points

Even if you're already a pro at EFT, follow along with me. I do it a bit differently than many practitioners do, so you might just learn something new or different. Let's start with the building blocks of this technique.

The first thing you need to know to use EFT is where you will actually be tapping on your face and body. You don't need to do anything with this yet; I just want you to understand where to tap when you're ready. While it's not important for you to understand which meridian (energy pathway) and associated emotions each point corresponds to, I do think it's interesting, so I'll briefly outline them for you now.

Tapping on a point creates a percussive effect that vibrates throughout the associated energy pathway and does the job of clearing. So while I want you to aim for the points, please know that this doesn't have to be done perfectly. As long as you're tapping in the general vicinity, you're golden!

Let's take this one step at a time.

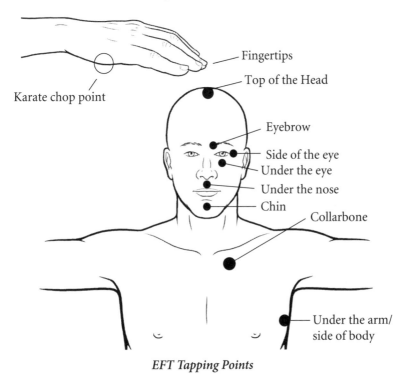

Fingertips

Top of the Head

Karate chop point

Eyebrow

Side of the eye

Under the eye

Under the nose

Chin

Collarbone

Under the arm/ side of body

EFT Tapping Points

(1) Karate chop point—*Tapping point:* The outside of your hand, about halfway between the bottom of your pinky and your wrist. This is where you would break a board if you were in martial arts.

Corresponds to: This point is commonly associated with overcoming self-sabotage and resistance to healing.

(2) Top of the head—*Tapping point:* This is smack dab in the middle of the top of your head.

Corresponds to: The governing meridian, a major energy pathway that runs down the back of the body, which is paired with another major meridian called the central meridian, which runs up the front of the body. These are two branches of the same energy pathway, representing the yin and yang of the body. They connect with the kidneys, heart, and brain.

(3) Eyebrow—*Tapping point:* The inside corner of the eye, right where the eyebrow starts.

Corresponds to: The bladder meridian, which deals with nervousness (connected to the nervous system), trauma, overwhelm, and hypersensitivity.

(4) Side of the eye—*Tapping point:* The outer corner of the eye, right on the bone. It's right inside your temple, closer to your eye.

Corresponds to: The gallbladder meridian, which deals with resentment, sadness, anger, and irritability.

(5) Under the eye—*Tapping point:* The top of the cheekbone, right under the eye.

Corresponds to: The stomach meridian, which deals primarily with worry.

(6) Under the nose—*Tapping point:* This is where a mustache would be if you had one.

Corresponds to: The governing meridian, which deals with shame and powerlessness.

(7) Chin—*Tapping point:* In the indentation on your chin, half-way between your bottom lip and the tip of your chin.

Corresponds to: The central meridian, a major energy pathway that runs up the front of the body, which is paired with another major meridian called the governing meridian, which runs down the back of the body. These are two branches of the same energy pathway, representing the yin and yang of the body. They connect with the kidneys, heart, and brain.

(8) Collarbone—*Tapping point:* Find where a man would tie a tie, then go out to the side an inch and drop directly under the collarbone.

Corresponds to: The kidney meridian, which deals primarily with fear.

(9) Under the arm/side of the body—*Tapping point:* This is where a bra band is, about four inches under the armpit on the side of the body.

Corresponds to: The spleen meridian, which deals with metabolizing thoughts and emotions and metabolizing life's experiences.

(10) Fingertips—*Tapping points:* The lower right-hand corner of each fingernail, where it meets the cuticle. You only need to tap on the fingertips of one hand.

Corresponds to: The thumb (lung meridian, linked to grief and depression), pointer finger (large intestine meridian, linked to letting go), middle finger (circulation-sex meridian, linked to anger), and pinky (heart meridian, linked to relationships and self love).

Note: The ring finger is not associated with any specific meridian but is included in the EFT process because it would be confusing to omit it.

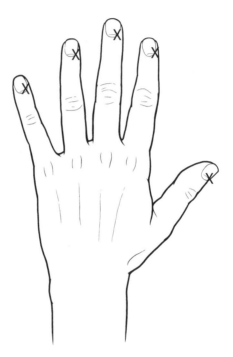

Fingertips Tapping Points

How to Tap

You can tap on just one side of the body or on both sides for each point. It works exactly the same, so do whatever feels most natural to you. I am a self-professed "lazy" tapper and use only one side of the face and body.

You want to aim for about 5–7 taps for each spot (please don't concentrate on this or count; it's just a general suggestion) and use medium pressure. Sometimes I have new tappers that tap so hard they end up in pain. If that happens to you, you are definitely tapping too firmly. If the points are mildly sore, it usually means the associated energy pathway has a lot of stuck energy and needs to be cleared, so go ahead and tap anyway. Use your fingertips to tap, versus your nails. Aside from that, you really can't go wrong with this technique, so just relax and go for it.

If you learned EFT before without the fingertip points, you simply learned a shortcut version. Some people skip certain tapping points to save time, but I always use all of the points to cover every energy pathway connected to the various organs, glands, muscles, and more. It's better to cover all of the bases than to try to save a few seconds.

How to Use Emotional Freedom Technique (EFT)

Now that you have the tapping points down, we're going to get into the clearing part. Just keep in mind that the ultimate goal of EFT is to (a) talk about the yucky feelings you have right now (either out loud or in your head) and then (b) tap at the same time to release them from your energy system. That's it. Easy! Talk as if you were telling me or a friend about how you feel and at the same time tap continuously through the points. I recommend talking out loud because it helps you stay focused on the task and it can also help move energy if done for productive reasons like with EFT. But if you are uncomfortable or unable to talk out loud, it's no biggie; just talk in your head. Don't get intimidated by putting a voice to your feelings. Most of us have a constant stream of thoughts in our head all the time about how we feel, why we might feel like this, and how we feel about feeling how we feel! The biggest obstacle people have in using this technique is not knowing what to say, but if you think about it, there is probably never a moment of silence in that head of yours. You already have all the words.

Note: I have some clients who are physically unable to use their hands to tap. If that's the case with you, simply close your eyes and imagine going through the tapping in the way I describe. Because everything (thoughts, emotions, your body) is just energy, we can actually move energy by visualizing the process. That might seem a little out there, but I assure you it works! Visualizing tapping is also my favorite middle-of-the-night anxiety-relief trick. If you can't physically tap because you don't want to wake your spouse, simply tap through the points and talk in your head. I use this method all the time with great success.

We're going to use a few easy steps as our guide as we learn EFT. This will give you a great foundation for using EFT on your own. In the appendix you will find a variety of tapping scripts that I've created to help guide you even further as you master using it for yourself.

1. Rate how you feel right now.
2. Create a set-up statement.
3. Use your set-up statement while tapping the karate chop point.
4. Tap through the rest of the points and vent.
5. Check in and repeat.
6. Wrap up your EFT session.

Step 1: Rate How You Feel Right Now

Start by giving a number from 1–10 (10 being the most intense) for how you feel now. Close your eyes for a moment and focus on how you are feeling. Focus on the anxiety temporarily. Let all the emotions and physical sensations come to your awareness for just a moment. For example, you might notice your heart racing and feeling unsettled, worried, and drained of energy.

Let your feelings come up to the surface. Remember, a huge reason that the feelings are stuck in the first place is because you've been pushing them down. Many clients tell me they are worried about feeling their feelings because they fear they'll be opening Pandora's box. But the truth is that you've already been feeling the feelings (hence the anxiety), so the only thing you are doing now is really allowing and acknowledging them so you can clear them. On a scale of 1–10, with 10 being the strongest, rate how intense this feeling is for you right *now*. If you can locate where you "feel" it in your body, make a mental note of that as well. For example, you might feel it as a pit in your stomach, an ache in your chest, or fuzziness in your head. If you don't feel it anywhere, that's fine too.

It doesn't matter what you're rating is when you start. You'll simply be using this number to gauge your progress as you clear.

Step 2: Create a Set-Up Statement

You will always start with what we call a *set-up statement* to describe your current feelings. There are two parts to this statement.

> *Even though* _____ *(describe how you feel right now),*
> *I can be okay anyway.*

Using this statement, you are acknowledging the feeling that you're dealing with but are sending a message that you can release it and move on anyway. The goal of being okay no matter what is a huge game-changer for healing anxiety, which is why I personally use the phrase about "being okay anyway" for the second part of the statement. But you'll see in just a minute that you can modify this in many different ways.

First Part of the Set-Up Statement

In the first part of your set-up statement, you want to use as much descriptive detail as possible to describe and "call out" the energy you focused on in step 1 so it can be cleared. You want to bring up the feelings and acknowledge them so they can be processed and moved out of your system.

> *Important Note:* An interesting phenomenon I've noticed over the years is that how a person feels about the anxiety is very indicative of what contributed to it in the first place. For example, try to identify your primary emotion about dealing with anxiety. Is it frustration or grief or anger? Whatever emotion(s) you resonate with most is likely the emotional energy that needs to be dealt with at a deep level in order to heal completely. That means that working with the primary feelings you have about living with anxiety can actually help to release the anxiety itself. We'll talk about how to use this trick in a more advanced way later (in chapter 7).

Here are some examples of what the first part might sound like; but please don't worry too much about how you describe how you feel, as long as it's true for you. That's what makes it work!

> Example: *Even though I feel so anxious and my heart is beating really fast and no matter what I do I can't stop worrying about everything, …*

Example: *Even though I'm so angry that I have this anxiety and it makes me feel sick to realize how much of my life I'm missing out on, ...*

Tip: Try to include a physical symptom and an emotional feeling in your set-up statement. Think of using this statement as a way to describe to your mind and body the problem you want to clear. Give your mind and body the details so they can help you release the problem.

Alternatives for the Second Part of the Set-Up Statement

The first part of your statement is telling your body and mind what you *don't* want, while the second part of the statement is essentially telling your mind and body what you *do* want. While my own go-to phrase for the second part of my statement is "I can be okay anyway," you can play around with alternatives and see what feels best for you. You basically just want to make sure you follow the following formula with whatever statement you create: tell your body what to let go of (first part) + tell your body what you want (second part).

Here are some examples of alternative phrases you could use for the second part of your set-up statement:

- *I completely love and accept myself.* This is the standard wording that's most commonly taught in EFT, but I almost never use it myself. It doesn't seem fitting for the things I typically tap for.
- *My body can relax now.* Getting the body to relax always has a positive impact on the nervous system.
- *I choose to release it.* This is an empowering statement that the body receives well.

- *I can heal anyway.* This one is beneficial because so many of us feel like our challenge is something we'll never be free from.

Once you have both parts of your set-up statement ready with something that's fitting for you, you can move on to the next step.

Step 3: Use Your Set-Up Statement While Tapping the Karate Chop Point

To begin the EFT process, say the entire set-up statement you put together three times in a row as you tap the karate chop point continuously. Use three or four fingers of one hand to tap the karate chop point of the other hand. Let's go over an example before you try it.

Example: *Even though I constantly worry about everything and it's making my heart race so much that I can't sleep or eat, I can be okay anyway.*

You can say the same statement three times exactly the same way, or you can change up the words so you're essentially saying the same thing in a different way. Here is an example of saying things differently:

Original: *Even though I constantly worry about everything and it's making my heart race so much that I can't sleep or eat, ...*

Alternate: *Even though I feel so anxious and my heart is beating really fast and no matter what I do I can't stop worrying about everything, ...*

Again, as long as whatever you are saying is an accurate statement of how you feel, any wording will work.

You can tap with your eyes open or closed. I always tap with mine closed because I find it easier to stay focused on how I feel and am less inclined to get distracted by my environment. If your mind wanders to the grocery list or some other thing, that's okay, but do your best to stick with whatever you're feeling. These feelings have likely been hanging out in your system for a long time, so it's better to temporarily focus on them in order to deal with them once and for all.

Let's try it now. Repeat your set-up statement three times as you tap your karate chop point continuously.

Example: *Even though I constantly worry about everything and it's making my heart race so much that I can't sleep or eat, I can be okay anyway.*

Now you're ready to move on and tap through the rest of the points.

Step 4: Tap Through the Rest of the Points and Vent

After tapping the karate chop point, simply tap through the rest of the points while you talk more about how you feel. This part of the process is the most fun. It's when I tell my clients, "Now you get to vent!" This means you get to let all your thoughts, feelings, and complaints out. Whatever you feel is fair game to talk and tap about. Try using a mix of emotional and physical sensations in your descriptions, meaning talk about how you feel emotionally and how it's making you feel physically (if you are feeling it in your physical body) and also how you feel *about* the anxiety. This doesn't have to be done in any particular order. In fact, it'll likely sound and feel like a bunch of random thoughts and feelings. That's exactly what it should be! As you tap and vent, allow whatever comes to mind to have a voice. Make sure you keep tapping while you talk about everything that is coming up for you even if it seems all over the place or feels silly. Your subconscious mind will often push forward thoughts, ideas, and connections in order to help you clear while using EFT. It's okay if they don't make logical sense or you can't figure out where they are coming from. Feelings and thoughts don't have to be analyzed or processed in a way that makes sense to you in order for you to resolve and release them. It's okay to allow things to come up and then just let them go.

It's important to remember that you are simply acknowledging the reality of your feelings in order to neutralize or release them. Saying these things out loud will not make them worse or create new feelings that weren't already there. Even if you tapped all day long saying "I'm scared of teddy bears," you would never end up with a fear of teddy bears. And if you were afraid of them in the first place, tapping would help clear that fear, so you're covered either way.

You don't need to use complete sentences as you tap. You can use words, phrases, or descriptions that make sense only to you. Focus on whatever is true about these feelings for you. That matters far more than the exact tapping points, how long you tap, or anything else. Just focus on venting about how you feel. An example of tapping through the rest of the points might look like the following, but remember to use your own phrases and feelings.

Top of the head—*I can't relax.*

Eyebrow—*I feel so anxious.*

Side of the eye—*I'm not even sure why I'm so anxious, but I'm frustrated!*

Under the eye—*I feel it in my _____.*

Under the nose—*It feels like* _____. (Example: *the world is ending* or *my stomach is always in knots.)*

Chin—*It feels like I'll never be normal and that is so scary.*

Collarbone—*I feel frozen.*

Under the arm/side of the body—*Grrrrrrr!* (Noises instead of words are good, too.)

Fingertip points—*I just wish I could feel better!*

Now continue tapping through the points again for a couple more rounds, from start to finish. Talk about how you feel and vent about whatever comes to mind again. It may be about the same things as before or new things may come up. Let it all out.

You are now ready to gauge your progress in the next step.

Step 5: Check In and Repeat

Take a break, open your eyes, take a deep breath or two, and check in with yourself. This gives the energy some time to process and shift. I sometimes shake off my hands or take a drink of water. You may be yawning, sighing, burping, suddenly exhausted, or feeling the energy shift in another way. If you don't, it's no problem. But a lot of people do sense the shifting.

Now close your eyes and tune back in to how you're feeling. Rate the intensity of the feeling on a scale of 1–10 again. Did the physical sensation or the emotional rating go down at all? Did it improve? If not, it's totally fine. Sometimes people will feel a shift with just a few rounds, so I'd like you to check. I am my own worst client though, as it often takes me many rounds of tapping and venting to feel a shift, and then after that it can take me a few hours or a few days to process all of that energy out of my system and actually start to feel better.

In any case, you'll want to repeat the whole process again from the beginning, either with the same words or different words—whatever feels natural. Make sure not to use your brain to censure this process of venting, as that will prevent you from really releasing what's there.

Even if you feel increased intensity after your first few rounds, don't worry. You may be surprised that any change is actually a really positive sign that the imbalanced energy is mobilizing and clearing. People will often feel a surge in an emotion or symptom as they tap. Again, this is simply just because we are bringing things to the surface that have been buried. Sometimes we'll kind of stir them up as part of the release process. Remember that because they were buried deep, you probably haven't been feeling the true feelings until now. They are just rising up close to the surface to be cleared. Yay! This is exactly what we want.

Do several more rounds, take breaks in between, and gauge if the energy is shifting. I often tap for anywhere from five to forty-five minutes, just to give you an idea of how long to use EFT each time. But it all depends on how you're feeling. If you start to feel great improvement, you don't need to tap for as long. This is a tool that you should integrate into your life as a way of making the shift from ignoring your feelings to helping them move out of your body. If you need help as you incorporate EFT into your life, remember that you have the tapping scripts in the appendix to support you.

Now the million-dollar question: How do you know if you're feeling better? Sometimes the shift isn't immediately obvious, especially if you're used to feeling no change at all. Do you feel like you're starting to calm down or feel even slightly better or more hopeful about your situation? Sometimes while clearing, improvement will manifest as you feeling the emotion less intensely in your body, feeling more optimistic, suddenly seeing things in a way you didn't before, or being more disconnected from that intense feeling you started with. If you did shift in a direction of feeling better from your first rounds, you'll want to simply keep tapping and venting. That's all there is to it.

Step 6: Wrap Up Your EFT Session

When you are feeling better or need to finish up with your tapping time, it's nice to wrap up with some positive tapping. Do not do this until the very end of your session though. Tapping and saying positive things all day will not help you release the emotions causing anxiety. Once in a while someone will tell me tapping didn't work for them. When I investigate further, I find out they've only been using the positive statements. We all know by now that trying to force ourselves to be positive doesn't work to cure anxiety. Tapping with only positive statements won't work either, as it defeats the purpose of EFT. Using positive statements is simply just a nice way to finish your session.

To close on a positive note, simply do one last round of tapping while focusing on some positive or calming phrases. It might look something like this:

Top of the head—*I'm okay.*

Eyebrow—*I can get past this.*

Side of the eye—*I want to feel better.*

Under the eye—*I'm feeling calmer now.*

Under the nose—*I rock!*

Chin—*I'm okay.*

Collarbone—*I'm okay.*

Under the arm/side of the body—*I think I can relax now.*

Fingertip points—*I'm okay.*

That's it! You can say anything that feels comforting to you. I usually mix up phrases, but it's perfectly okay to repeat the same positive phrase, such as *I'm okay*, over and over. There are no rules here.

Additional Tapping Techniques to Help You Deal With Your Feelings

Here are some additional ideas for using various methods of tapping. All of these can be used in addition to EFT or as a supplement to it.

Use EFT Inconspicuously or in Public

If you're in a place where you can't tap out in the open, simply put your hand in an inconspicuous place (such as under a table at a restaurant) and use only the karate chop and fingertip points from EFT. In this kind of situation, you don't even need to do the set-up statement and phrases—just tap, tap, tap.

Use Subconscious Tapping

This is my favorite trick I created while learning to use EFT. Sometimes I found myself not able to identify how I felt or what was making me anxious. If you can relate, here's something fun to try. I use this when I'm feeling lost and am not sure what to say or where to start. Calling on the subconscious mind to help is a great way to release yucky energy, even if we don't know exactly what needs to be cleared. Remember, the subconscious mind knows everything—which is scary and awesome at the same time!

To begin, use this set-up statement: *Even though I have no idea what this anxiety is about, I give my subconscious permission to release it anyway.*

While tapping on the rest of the points, focus on the anxiety itself as you vent. (Include any emotions or thoughts you have about it just as you normally would.) Every few tapping points, add in this phrase: *I don't know what's making me anxious, but my subconscious does.*

Just keep tapping in that way. This will trigger your subconscious to pull up whatever information needs to be cleared, even if you don't ever know what it is.

Add This Additional Powerful EFT Point

About halfway down the top of the hand, in between the pinky and ring fingers, there is a point that corresponds to the triple warmer meridian. As you know, this meridian governs the fight, flight, or freeze response. This point is often referred to as the gamut point in EFT, but you'll also recognize it as the Panic Point from chapter 4. Because it's located right along the triple warmer meridian line, we use it as a tool for neutralizing panic and fear.

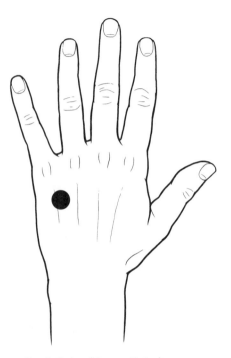

Panic Point (Gamut Point)

Adding this point to your EFT process, along with a seemingly silly little routine of eye movements, head shifting, and humming, helps engage the right and left hemispheres of the brain. This process has been shown to be extremely useful in releasing and processing old feelings and traumas. It's a little confusing to learn when you're first figuring out the basics, which is why I didn't introduce it earlier. But I do want you to add this point and see if it helps you feel better faster. It often does! This point will come after the last fingertip tapping point (the pinky) and before you go back to the karate chop point. I don't use it every single time but add it more intuitively, or simply just when I remember to do so! When you get to the gamut point in your tapping routine, do the following as you continue to tap on it:

Close your eyes, open your eyes, shift your eyes down and to the right (don't move your head), shift your eyes down and to the left (don't move your head), roll your eyes in a big circle in front of you, then roll them in the other direction, hum a few seconds of a song (anything will do!), count to five quickly out loud (1, 2, 3, 4, 5), and then hum for a few more seconds. Again, you'll then just move on to the karate chop point and keep tapping as you normally would from there.

It may seem like a lot right now, but you'll be surprised how quickly you memorize it after using it several times.

Use Chakra Tapping

Once I got the hang of EFT, I really loved it. I also made a discovery for my own healing through using it. I played around with different ideas on how to use tapping and discovered that if I tapped on points that corresponded to chakras instead of meridians (used in EFT), things would often change faster or differently! This is when I tweaked EFT and created a process that I call *Chakra Tapping*. For Chakra Tapping, I use the exact same format as in EFT, but instead of EFT points, I use chakra tapping points.

As we discussed in chapter 1, chakras are spinning energy centers in the body. There are seven main chakras throughout the body. Chakras store old stories in the body. The energies of these stories are directly tied to early childhood programming and conditioning. Each chakra governs a different area of the physical body. Energy imbalances in the chakras often show up as symptoms in the related physical area. That's why tapping on the points that correspond to each chakra can be so beneficial! EFT and Chakra Tapping can be used interchangeably. If you aren't getting enough of a shift from one set of points, switch to the other!

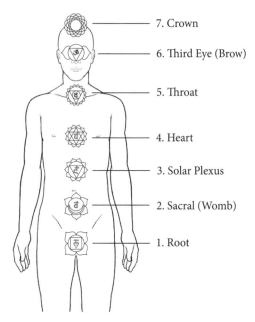

The Seven Main Chakras

Crown (Seventh) Chakra Tapping Point—Top of the head

Third Eye or Brow (Sixth) Chakra Tapping Point—In between the eyebrows

Throat (Fifth) Chakra Tapping Point—Front of the throat

Heart (Fourth) Chakra Tapping Point—In the middle of the chest

Solar Plexus (Third) Chakra Tapping Point—Right under the sternum at your solar plexus

Sacral (Second) Chakra Tapping Point—Just below the belly button

Root (First) Chakra Tapping Point—Top of your thighs (Pat them like you're calling a puppy up on your lap.)

To use Chakra Tapping, you'll follow the exact same process as you did with EFT, but after the karate chop point, start rotating through the chakra points—starting from the crown chakra down to your root chakra and then back to the karate chop point.

Use Tapping Shortcuts

Tapping is so easy that you should be able to use it quickly and without any preparation, but I understand that being anxious can make everything feel overwhelming. So here are a few shortcuts you can use if you ever find yourself feeling too anxious to do the full tapping routine.

Use Only the Collarbone Point: Tap only the collarbone point, which is linked to the kidney meridian (associated primarily with the emotion of fear). This point is very powerful on its own, and in a pinch, it may help provide you with relief without doing the entire EFT process. You can do this for anywhere from a few times to several minutes.

Clear the Solar Plexus Chakra: Tapping on just the solar plexus chakra point is great for anxiety, especially since that chakra is related to feeling powerless or unsafe. Clearing imbalances in this area can help you to feel more empowered and confident. Use solar plexus tapping for a few minutes at a time.

Skip the Set-Up Statement: Skipping the set-up statement is okay to do from time to time, especially if it's stopping you from using EFT when you're very anxious.

Tap without Talking: If you're feeling very upset, it's okay to tap through the points without saying anything. The talking, or venting, part of the process helps to bring up suppressed emotions. However, if you're already crying or very upset about something in particular, those emotions are probably already at the surface! You don't need to talk out loud and say, "I'm so upset, I can't stop crying." Just allow yourself to feel yucky and tap, tap, tap through all the points until you're feeling better.

Thymus Tapping: While tapping the thymus gland (like you learned in chapter 1) isn't part of EFT, I often use it as a shortcut to dealing with my feelings. I'm sure you can see by now that I'm a big fan of any kind of tapping to release stuck energy! In the same way you might just use the karate chop point or the collarbone point, you can tap on your thymus gland to help calm your emotions.

Work with Feelings about Anxiety: Remember, focusing on how you feel *about* the anxiety while using EFT or Chakra Tapping is a great way to start releasing it. Even if you don't address the anxiety itself, but rather all of your frustration, sadness, and hopelessness *about* it, you'll make some great progress toward feeling better.

The more you practice tapping, the more ways you'll find to use it. The general rule I'd like you to follow is the one I make for my clients, which I alluded to earlier. If you're feeling bad, use tapping! Tapping even for just a few minutes at a time will get you feeling better much faster than if you just sit there feeling miserable. Remember, you can use the tapping scripts in the appendix to help guide you as well.

You have now successfully gained the tools you need to deal with feelings that you've been struggling with from day to day. This is amazing because now you'll never have to ignore and suppress them again. Woohoo!

While using EFT and Chakra Tapping in the way I just taught you can be very helpful first steps, you're now ready to get to the root of the anxiety, identify what caused it in the first place, and release them from your body forever. You'll be re-visiting your past and delving into it a bit deeper in the next chapter.

Summary

Learning to deal with our feelings is an essential part of healing from anxiety and preventing it from coming back. *Not* dealing with our feelings is what helped us get to this place. That's why we want to undo that old pattern. Dealing with our feelings in the present moment is actually quite straightforward: we need to allow ourselves to feel the emotions coming up while using tools to help move them out.

EFT and Chakra Tapping are great techniques to help move emotional energy out of the system. They are effective and easy to use. All you have to do is talk about your feelings (aka vent!) and tap on various points at the same time. Tap and talk—that's it. Practice these techniques when you are feeling difficult emotions and you will be well on your way to emotional healing.

Section III

* * * * * * * * * * * * * * *

Address the Root
of Anxiety

* * * * * * * * * * * * * * * *

Chapter Six

Release Stuck Emotions

You've already learned several excellent ways to use tapping to deal with your feelings as they come up. That will go a long way toward helping you feel better *now* and preventing anxiety in the future. But as I see it, the core root of anxiety is emotional energy that is stuck in the body due to being suppressed, typically over a period of many years. That's why, in addition to dealing with our current feelings, we need to release stuck emotions from the past that we've been carrying. Otherwise, those emotions will stay lodged in our body and may be felt permanently in the form of anxiety.

In this chapter we'll be learning exactly how old emotions (that we never dealt with) can get stuck in the body long after we experience them, how they affect our wellbeing, and how to go back and release them in order to relax and heal. You'll be learning how to do this by using an advanced EFT method and learning a new technique called Thymus Test and Tap (TTT).

If stuffing emotions is a pattern for you, this might be the first time you've ever experienced what it's like not to have the burden of all those extra emotions from the past stuck in your body. You're in for a serious treat!

Understanding Trauma

Many people understand that trauma can lead to lasting emotional (and physical) challenges. Trauma is often thought of as abuse, neglect, an accident, or a catastrophe, but trauma is essentially *any* deeply distressing or disturbing experience, no matter how big or small it seems. This means that anything from a death in the family to something hurtful your friend said to you on the playground in elementary school could be considered trauma. Recall from when you learned about EFT in chapter 5 that it's not necessarily what happened to you but rather how your body's energy system reacted to an experience that leads to the end result. This means that anything can be *traumatizing*, even if we wouldn't necessarily consider it *traumatic*. That's why so many people come to me with anxiety saying, "I don't understand why I have this! Nothing *that bad* has ever happened to me." And often, "I've talked about all my memories and feelings in therapy for years and it isn't helping enough." Addressing the energy system in conjunction with traumatic memories and emotions can make all the difference in successfully healing from them.

This concept of traumatizing experiences is very important to understand because a lot of people make the mistake of ignoring their past due to the belief that "others had it worse than them" or they "haven't experienced enough trauma to cause *this* much anxiety." But sometimes the experiences from life that stick with us are the ones that felt like no big deal in relationship to what we normally think of as traumatic.

When something really difficult and obviously traumatic happens to us, we typically seek help, talk to our friends about it, and more. But when it feels small or insignificant, we brush it off as no big deal and don't recognize or acknowledge how much it has impacted us.

When we have a negative reaction to an experience and then don't process and release emotions we are feeling, they can become lodged in the body. This can happen whether an experience seemed big and traumatic or like almost nothing. Either way, we end up with the same result: a whole lot of emotional energy stuck in a place where it shouldn't be—in us.

During our work with emotional energy throughout this book, let's agree not to write anything off as "too small" to address. Any emotions that are stuck in the body and having a negative impact on our lives need to be released.

Emotional Triggers

For each event or experience in your life, you may have a specific feeling (or many feelings) associated with the memory. Think back to a positive experience in your life. Do you feel that in your body? Are you relaxed, happy, or content? Now think back to a difficult experience. Do you feel tense or anxious or even some negative physical symptoms? Those different feelings are probably in alignment with whatever was going on at the time. Positive memories of the past are nice to keep around and recall, but emotions around something stressful or upsetting that are stored in the body only create "triggers" for anxiety. A trigger happens when our current situation reminds us of a past experience and activates old emotions stored in the body. This reignites the negative feelings from the past.

Neuroscientist Candace Pert wrote the following in her groundbreaking book *Molecules of Emotion:* "Emotional memory is stored in many places in the body, not just or even primarily in the brain....I think unexpressed emotions are literally lodged in the body. The real true emotions that need to be expressed are in the body, trying to move up and be expressed and thereby integrated, made whole, and healed."[5] Simply put, unexpressed emotions from experiences can get stuck in the body at the level of cellular memory.

The simple explanation for this is that if you don't acknowledge and fully feel your emotions, they can get lodged or stuck in your body. Emotions that are stuffed down instead of acknowledged and allowed can continually trigger you until you let them go.

The big challenge you might have had up until now is that, like almost all of my clients, you don't know what the heck is triggering the anxiety. In other words, you have no idea what emotions are stuck in your body, what experiences those emotions originated in, or why or when they get activated. But don't worry, we are going to solve that problem completely in this chapter. We'll also discuss how to prevent emotions from getting stuck in the future.

It's important to know that everyone has emotions stuck in their body—and a lot of them. But that's totally normal and not all of them are affecting you negatively. Now you're going to learn a technique I created to help you identify which emotions to release even if you have no idea how the heck they got there.

I bet you're less anxious already just knowing that, right?

Use Thymus Test and Tap (TTT) to Release Stuck Emotions

Using a technique called Thymus Test and Tap (TTT), you're going to release individual emotions lodged in your body. These emotions may have gotten stuck in your body at any time in your life and may be unrelated to one another. They can be

---

5. Candace B. Pert, PhD, *Molecules of Emotion* (New York: Simon & Schuster, 1999), http://candacepert.com/where-do-you-store-your-emotions/.

stored anywhere in your body, can be stuck along with other emotions, and can be accessed and cleared individually even with almost no knowledge or information about them.

TTT utilizes the powerful thymus gland—the master gland of the body's immune system—to clear stuck emotional energy throughout the body. The thymus gland is located near the heart in the emotional energy center of the body (see the illustration on page 32) and is often referred to as the "heart's protector." It is the first thing in the body that is energetically affected by emotions. From an energetic perspective, the thymus gland regulates the energy flow throughout your entire body. This gland is affected most by feeling unsafe, unprotected, or attacked by life or others. It makes perfect sense why it would play such an important role in healing anxiety, doesn't it?

The thymus gland is the star of this technique because it is connected to the rest of the body's energy system and is so powerful. By tapping the thymus gland, almost any block or imbalance in the system can be cleared.

While there are many techniques out there to help us release emotions, TTT allows us to process and release individual emotions while *also* rebalancing the immune system, nervous system, and heart field energy.

To help you release stuck emotions, you'll use a simple two-part process. First, you'll need to identify the actual emotions that are stuck in your body. Then you'll use a simple thymus-tapping procedure to release them.

Let's discuss the first thing I bet you're wondering about: *How in the world am I going to know what specific emotions are stuck in my body?* Don't worry, I've got you covered. Using a list of unprocessed emotions that I created (see page 120), I'm going to show you how to identify which emotions you need to release using a few different methods. You can choose whatever method works best for you. You only need to use one of them.

This list was made based on my analysis of common emotions that tend to remain in the body long after an experience is over. I left extra spots on the list so that if there are emotions you resonate with that I didn't include, you can add them yourself.

The process you are about to learn includes identifying an emotion and then releasing it, identifying another emotion and releasing it, and so on. You'll keep going through this two-part process for your entire releasing session.

I want to warn you that this isn't a one-time process, because everyone has hundreds or more emotions stuck in their body. This is totally normal and there is no need to worry if you feel like you have more stuck emotions than years you've lived. I've never kept track, but I bet I've done hundreds of sessions for myself using this technique alone. The great part is that you'll probably be pretty excited to do them since this process is so easy and fun!

Releasing even a couple emotions can make a big difference in how you feel, so think of this as a marathon, not a sprint. A single emotion that you let go of can clear a huge amount of anxiety, so don't underestimate the power of each release.

Thymus Test and Tap (TTT) Technique

Let's do this together now, step by step.

Step 1: Identify the Stuck Emotions (One at a Time)

You'll begin by using a list of unprocessed emotions I compiled (see chart), along with one of the techniques I'll outline next, to identify which feelings are stuck in your body. Remember, you'll be identifying and clearing one emotion at a time.

Option A: Identify an Emotion Using Muscle Testing: The first and best way to identify old emotions is to use your superpower of muscle testing. Remember, your subconscious mind is like a recorder. It knows exactly what old feelings may still be linked to the unprocessed experience you are working with. It's a common practice among certain types of practitioners to utilize muscle testing as a way to identify imbalances in the body. Homeopathic doctors and naturopaths often use lists of various bacteria and viruses along with muscle testing to detect which microbes are affecting their patients. Integrative nutritionists often use food frequency lists or vials along with muscle testing to discover what their clients are allergic to. For the TTT technique, you're going to be using the same idea/method and focusing on a list of emotions to find out which ones are stuck in your body.

To muscle-test which emotions are stuck in your body, you can use the Standing Test or the O-Ring Test, which you learned in chapter 3. Ask your body out loud or in your head, *Can I release an emotion on this list that's contributing to anxiety?* You can alter the wording of this question to whatever is comfortable for you. It doesn't have to be worded exactly as I've suggested. I sometimes ask, *Is there a stuck emotion causing anxiety that my body wants to let go of?*

| Thymus Test and Tap (TTT) Unprocessed Emotions ||
Section 1	*Section 2*
Abandoned	Defensive
Attacked	Failure
Berated	Frustrated
Betrayed	Heavy
Criticized	Helpless
Fearful	Hopeless
Grief-stricken	Impatient
Hated	Insecure
Intimidated	Out of control
Judged	Panicked
Uneasy	Powerless
Worthless	Shocked
Section 3	*Section 4*
Angry	Alone
Blamed	Bullied
Conflicted	Despair
Confused	Disappointed
Devastated	Discarded
Disgusted	Excluded
Guilty	Lonely
Hurt	Overwhelmed
Indecisiveness	Regretful
Nervous	Shamed
Resentful	Undeserving
Unsafe	Unsupported
Worried	

Note: It is totally normal for the exact same emotion to come up multiple times. The reason for this is because you can have that emotion stuck in your body from different times in your life. For instance, you might have sadness stuck in your body from when your pet hamster died when you were ten. You might also have it stuck from when you broke up with a partner at age twenty-five. In addition, we all have a tendency to feel certain feelings and therefore are more likely to have those stuck than others. For example, when you get in an argument with a loved one, you might tend to feel sadness more than anger, while someone else might go straight to anger first.

You will almost certainly get a "yes" from your body for releasing emotions contributing to anxiety. If you get a "no," it may be a rare instance where the timing to work on yourself is just not right. You may be rushed or dehydrated or just need to be in a better space. You can check again in a few hours or the next day.

Remember, for the Standing Test, a sway forward means "yes" from your body and a sway backward means "no." For the O-Ring Test, a "yes" is when your "O" stays strong and sealed together, while a "no" is when it breaks apart fairly easily.

If you get a "yes" to your first question, then ask, *Is it [the stuck emotion] in section 1?* If you get a "no," you'll know that the stuck emotion is in one of the other sections on the list, so you can ask about each of those sections until you get a "yes." Then read each emotion in the section you've identified one by one, asking your body, *Is it _____?* Do this until you get a "yes." If you want to try a shortcut, glance at the chart and see what stands out to you. Then muscle-test those individual emotions first to see if they are the one(s) your body is looking for.

Option B: Identify an Emotion by Running Your Finger over the List: Another great way to identify the emotions your body wants to release is to use a process where you let your body intuitively guide you. I consider this a form of muscle testing, but it's a bit more relaxed. Close your eyes and very gently swirl your pointer finger all over the list of unprocessed emotions. If you do this very, very lightly, you might feel your finger "stick" or slow down a little bit over the emotion that your body resonates with and wants to release right now. You might also just get a sense of when you want to stop. Your body is actually picking up on the right emotions for you. This may feel like a sloppy way of choosing emotions, but I actually find it quite accurate!

Let's pause here while you identify your first stuck emotion using either option A or option B.

> *Note:* While "anxiety" appears on pretty much every other list of emotions that I've seen out there, it does not appear on mine. By now you should understand that anxiety is not an emotion but is the end result of what happens when we don't allow and express our emotions.

Step 2: Discover More About the Emotion (Optional)

In some cases, it is helpful for the body's releasing process if you know a bit more information about the emotion you just identified, such as the age and event that created the stuck emotion in the first place. It won't be necessary for you to learn more about the majority of the emotions you identify, but for the ones that your body does want you to dig a bit deeper with, it's worth taking the time. The only way to know for sure which emotions to get information about is to ask the body through muscle testing. The importance of finding out more about some emotions lies in the body wanting you to finally acknowledge and honor the emotion so it can feel and release it as it should have originally.

The reason I have this as an optional step is that I like to keep things as simple as possible when teaching a technique. However, if you feel up for this, I strongly advise giving it a try. This extra step, which gives your body the opportunity to help you understand the origin of the emotion, may help you process at a deeper level, resulting in greater and faster improvement. Again, we're giving your body the chance to tell us if it would be beneficial to know more, but it won't apply to every emotion. Simply use muscle testing to ask your body, *Would it be beneficial to know more about this emotion?* If you get a "yes," you may want to find out what age the emotion is stuck from. Ask via muscle testing, *Did this emotion get stuck from an event between the ages of 0 and 20?* If you get a "yes," narrow it down further until you get a specific age. If you get a "no," ask if the emotion got stuck between the ages of 20 and 40, and so on.

Once you find the age, you can ask again, *Would it be beneficial to know more about this emotion?* If you get a "yes," it's all about guessing—unless of course you remember something significant from that age, such as a relationship breakup, a move, a health issue, etc. Try to think in terms of what you were doing during that time in your life and see if that helps trigger anything. Remember, you are not necessarily looking for an obviously traumatic experience. If you can think of something, ask your body questions to get confirmation. For example, *Is this emotion stuck from _____ (insert the event you recall)?*

If you get a "yes," you can stop and move on to step 3, where you'll release the emotion. If you get a "no," keep guessing. You could also ask about a certain person, a place, and more. Here are some examples: *Is this stuck emotion related to Mom? Is this stuck emotion related to when I lived in that moldy apartment? Is this stuck emotion related to school?*

Step 3: Release the Emotion

Now you're ready to tap your thymus to release this emotion from your body. To release the emotion, simply tap seven times firmly over your thymus gland with the fingertips of one hand. As you do this, just hold the intention of clearing or tapping that emotion out of your system and make sure you breathe.

If you've used other techniques and approaches, you may be accustomed to analyzing your emotions from the past. Human beings usually desire some kind of understanding before they can let go of something. However, unless your body has specifically asked for you to know more (in step 2), you can just let the emotion go. Personally, I just tap, release, and move on! But I do have clients who have certain rituals they do as they release. Some people find it nice to say something while they perform the tapping. If you wish, you could repeat the word *clearing* or *releasing* as you tap. I have clients who take deep yogic breaths, hum, repeat the words *thank you*, and more while they tap. But again, I'm a "tap and be done" kind of person, so do whatever feels natural to you.

Step 4: Repeat the Process

After releasing each emotion, simply go back to step 1 and start over.

Releasing stuck emotions can't be done all at one time in an hour, a day, or even a week. This is something you do little by little. After every five to ten emotions that you release, take a little break.

You can use your intuition to know when to stop and wait until the next session to do more, or you can ask via muscle testing (*Is it beneficial for me to continue using TTT?*). You'll get a "no" from your body with muscle testing when it's time to stop. Most people can clear 10–30 emotions at a time, but if you're feeling really tired or don't wish to continue for whatever reason, it's best to slow down or wait a day or two.

Step 5: Install Positive Emotions

Just as we can use TTT to clear unwanted emotions, we can use it to install positive emotions as well. Installing positive emotions is equivalent to doing a positive round of tapping when we're wrapping up an EFT session (from chapter 5). The practice of installing positive emotions will enhance the work you're doing by giving your body positive emotions to put in the place of the ones you've released. Installing positive energy is a nice way to complete the healing process in the body. Using the list of positive emotions shown here, you will be identifying and installing them one by one. Feel free to add additional positive emotions to the list.

I like to install 3–5 positive emotions at the end of every TTT session. You can do this by muscle-testing to find the most beneficial emotions or simply installing a few that pop out to you or resonate with you.

Thymus Test and Tap (TTT) Positive Emotions	
Section 1	*Section 2*
Able	Comforted
Abundant	Connected
Accepted	Content
Accepting	Decisive
Adaptable	Deserving
Appreciated	Empowered
Assertive	Encouraged
At ease	Energetic
Brave	Flowing
Inspired	Forgiven
Joyful	Free
Light	Grounded
Protected	Happy
Reassured	Loved
Section 3	*Section 4*
Acknowledged	Calm
Empowered	Centered
Grateful	Confident
Important	Healed
Included	Hopeful
Independent	Open
Relaxed	Optimistic
Secure	Peaceful
Soothed	Positive
Strong	Trusting
Supported	Valued
Understood	Willing

If you are muscle testing, ask your body this question: *Is there a positive feeling on this list that would be beneficial for me to install now?* If you get a "yes," go to the next question: *Is it in section 1?* If you get a "no," then you'll know it's in one of the other sections on the list and can then ask about each of those sections until you get a "yes." Then read each emotion in the section you've identified one by one, asking your body, *Is it _____?* Do this until you get a "yes."

Once you've identified the emotion you want to install, tap seven times firmly over your thymus gland with the fingertips of one hand. Hold the intention that you're tapping that positive energy into your thymus gland and sending a force of the positive energy throughout your system. As you do this, imagine the positive word or focus on the positive feeling. Take a few deep breaths.

How and Why Thymus Test and Tap (TTT) Works

Let's talk about how and why this method works so you understand what's happening in your body. The tapping creates a percussive effect that sends a force of energy through your thymus gland to clear the emotional energy that is creating a block or imbalance, wherever it is in your system. You don't need to know where the block or imbalance is located, which is great. Your intention to release it is also helping to clear it. You are acknowledging the feeling while giving your body permission to let it go. At the same time that you are tapping your thymus gland to release the emotion, you are also rebalancing and strengthening your system, allowing it to recover from the imbalance and integrate the healing process.

You may find that you yawn, sigh, burp, or feel the energy shift in some other way. If you don't, don't worry at all. The process works either way.

Additional Ways to Use Thymus Test and Tap (TTT)

TTT can be used for all different kinds of emotional clearing. In addition to using it in the way I just taught you (by focusing on emotions causing anxiety), you can also approach clearing anxiety in some other interesting ways.

Focus on Specific Aspects of Anxiety

Sometimes I'll look at someone's big-picture "anxiety story" (what they are telling me they already know about causes and triggers) and use TTT to work on different aspects of that. Here are some examples on how I've done that with clients.

Mallory was triggered every time she had to see her stepmom, Nancy, at a family function or even just talk to her on the phone. She had never had a good relationship with her, and things seemed to get worse into her adulthood. So instead of using TTT only for anxiety in general, we decided to apply it more specifically to her reaction to her stepmom. We used muscle testing to identify "emotions linked to or triggered by Nancy." When we did this, Mallory became much less reactive to Nancy, and even when Mallory did get triggered, she found it much easier to calm down and move on now that we had worked specifically with energy related to Nancy. If you have a specific person or people in your life whom you've noticed the anxiety gets triggered around, using TTT for these different aspects could be a huge help.

Steve was terrified to drive at night. He had a few inklings why, which were related to specific memories from his past. (You'll be learning how to deal with specific memories in the next chapter.) However, we weren't getting a huge shift from approaching it that way. But when we added in releasing emotions related to the following specific aspects of driving at night, everything started to improve: "emotions triggered in cars," "emotions related to the dark," "emotions linked to eyes." Taking your bigger picture story and then breaking it down into parts, or aspects, might just give you a major breakthrough.

There is no set formula for figuring out what specific aspects of the bigger picture to clear emotions around, but the things you could use TTT for are pretty much endless. Here are a few general ideas for you. Writing a quick summary paragraph of your own situation in the way that I did with my examples may help you break it down into smaller things you could apply TTT to.

You could use TTT to release old emotions linked to the following:

- A specific person (Mom, Dad, etc.)
- A time period in your life (high school, first job, etc.)
- A specific job (*when I worked at* _____)
- A theme (such as intimate relationships)
- An activity that triggers anxiety (like travel, public speaking, going to the doctor, etc.)
- A pattern that's hard for you to break (self-sabotage, being critical, etc.)
- A specific place (such as *my childhood home*)
- A physical symptom (digestive issues, migraines, etc.)
- A specific age (age ten, age thirty-seven, etc.)

You don't need to be particularly organized or strategic here. Just pick some different ideas from the list I provided and give it a try. Starting with what you know triggers you now is an excellent place to start.

Use TTT While Triggered

TTT is a great tool when you are in the midst of a crisis. If you can identify and release emotions during times of intense anxiety, you can clear some of the root cause right there and then. By doing this, you'll be clearing emotions being triggered from the past, which will make it less likely that they'll be an issue in the future. Using muscle testing, ask, *Can I find and release an emotion being triggered right now?* Release what you find. Then repeat the process until you've cleared them all.

Use TTT after Panic Attacks

One of the best times to use TTT is after an "incident" such as a panic attack. If you can identify the emotions that were triggered, you can clean them up to limit the chances of experiencing another similar situation. Years ago, I had a terrible panic attack when I took my wife to urgent care when she had a terrible cold. It was very strange, as I had been through so many medical situations myself without any issues. As they took her blood pressure, I got dizzy and had to run into the bathroom to throw up. A similar situation happened again at a later time. I was puzzled! But using TTT, I released emotions that were triggered by those events, and they never happened again. Phew!

Using muscle testing, ask, *Can I find and release an emotion that triggered _____ (describe the event, like "that panic attack at the doctor's office last week")?* Release what you find. Then repeat the process until you've cleared them all.

Install Positive Emotions

Positive feelings should be installed after you've released negative emotions, but I also like to use this method when I'm feeling low or off and want an emotional boost. Simply ask your body through muscle testing or intuitively what emotions you can install to help boost your body.

Prevent New Emotions From Getting Stuck

Now that you understand how emotions get lodged in your body, let's discuss a few easy strategies to prevent that from happening.

The first thing is to stay aware of and more tuned in to how you're feeling. Remember that these emotions get stuck because we suppress them. While we don't always suppress our feelings consciously, we often do. You'll see this if you pay close attention to how you're feeling more often. When you notice your feelings, commit to allowing yourself to feel your feelings and acknowledge your emotions instead of talking yourself out of them. Don't tell yourself "It's no big deal!" if it really is. Acknowledge how you're feeling and accept it, even if it doesn't make logical sense to you or you don't like it. It won't hurt you to feel how you feel. If we can master allowing ourselves to feel how we feel without resistance or judgment, we can truly stop the cycle of stuffed—and stuck—emotions.

Using the techniques you already know will really help too. In addition to using TTT during difficult moments, you can also do a few rounds of EFT to help move that energy out.

You can also practice the techniques from chapter 4, which will help your body calm down instead of getting stuck in fight, flight, or freeze mode.

You don't need to use all of my suggestions. Just simply pick one and use it for a few minutes when you need it. That's more than enough to create the healthy habit of releasing emotions instead of suppressing them.

When people learn about stuck emotions, they sometimes start fearing that every emotion they feel will get stuck in their body and cause anxiety. This is not true at all. You've felt millions of emotions in your life and not all of them got stuck. In addition, not every emotion that is still with you is causing anxiety. There's no need to be paranoid about your emotions. The important thing is that you become more aware of and change the general pattern you've had of suppressing your emotions. A few emotions here and there that you don't deal with in the healthiest way is not going to make or break you—I promise!

Summary

Dealing with our feelings as they arise is essential for working with anxiety, but we also need to dig deeper and clear emotions from the past that may be stuck in the body. Emotions, when not properly acknowledged and processed, can get lodged in the body. These emotions can be felt all the time and can be huge triggers for anxiety, even when we're not aware that they're there and don't know what they are or how they got stuck.

Thymus Tap and Test (TTT) is an excellent technique for releasing those stuck emotions and alleviating anxiety. It can be used in so many ways that the sky really is the limit!

You now have a variety of tools you can use to prevent emotions from getting stuck in the future: calming and retraining techniques (to address the fight, flight, or freeze response), EFT, and TTT.

* * * * * * * * * * * * * *

Chapter Seven

Clear Unprocessed Experiences from the Past

With TTT, we've been working with individual emotions stuck in the body. Although it's possible that some of the emotions you'll find using TTT will be related to each other (from the same experience), it's likely a lot of them are just floating around from hundreds of different time periods in your life. Identifying and releasing individual emotions is a great way to release anxiety. Next, I'm going to teach you another approach so you can keep peeling back those emotional layers and continue to heal.

In this chapter we'll be learning how to deal with memories from your past as a whole, which I call *unprocessed experiences*. I guarantee that these experiences are probably triggering you, even if they seem "small." Most importantly, I'm going to teach you exactly how to clear them with an advanced (but still super easy!) EFT method.

Defining Unprocessed Experiences

Any disturbing or distressing event or emotional experience from your life that you have not acknowledged, processed, and released from your body could still be affecting you negatively today. This is what I call an unprocessed experience. Simply put, it means that you are still carrying the energy of a difficult experience from your past. In addition to clearing individual emotions with TTT, working with a memory or past experience as a whole is another excellent way to effectively clear anxiety.

Here's a metaphor to help you understand how unprocessed experiences get created and how they might trigger anxiety. Imagine there is a little glass capsule in your body. When you have an upsetting experience and don't process and release the energy associated with it, all of the details associated with the experience get stored in that capsule and remain there: emotions, images, scents, colors, sounds, etc. When anything you are currently experiencing reminds you of or matches the details stored inside that capsule, that unprocessed experience can get triggered, activating it in your body. That's when you can feel anxious, recalling memories or details of the past (although this may be totally subconscious) and related emotions that have been percolating beneath the surface.

An unprocessed experience can be an obvious event from your past (such as the death of a friend or family member) or something seemingly small (such as missing your friend's birthday party because you had the flu). Energy from any event can become stuck in the body and create anxiety. Here are some characteristics of unprocessed experiences:

- Any event that you have not **acknowledged** means you most likely said to yourself in some way, even if subconsciously, "Oh, that was no big deal!" when you really were feeling like, "Whoa, this *feels* like a big deal (even if it's silly)!"

- Any event that you have not **processed** means that you don't yet understand it or have not yet come to peace with not understanding it—and it remains unfinished with your spirit.

- Any event that you have not **released** means that because you have not acknowledged and processed it, it might still be stored in your body. If this is true for you, you will most likely feel a "charge" when you recall it. This could show up as a knot in your stomach, tension in your chest, tears in your eyes, a racing heart, sweaty hands, and more.

A good way to determine if an experience of yours is unprocessed is to see if you feel an emotional "charge" when you think about the memory. This charge can be any feeling, but typically it's a pit in your stomach, tightness in your chest, a nervous feeling, and so on. Any uncomfortable sensation when you recall a memory is an indicator that there's still unprocessed energy there. Think of this energy or "charge" as the *bzzzt* we talked about earlier that happens in the energy system. It's essentially an energy imbalance in relationship to the experience or memory you have.

Let's look at Jesse's story to understand how these experiences affect us. Jesse was a client of mine in his early twenties. When he was five, he was the smallest kid in the class and was made fun of incessantly for it. It really affected him and his ability to form healthy friendships as he got older. Jesse had several upsetting memories but one particularly strong memory of being surrounded by three girls in his class who were calling him "shorty" and "baby." He still felt a pit in his stomach when he thought about it. He didn't want to tell anyone about this experience, so he kept it to himself. Plus, he had a couple good friends now who couldn't have cared less about his size, so he tried to focus on that.

Because he had never dealt with that experience from his youth, it remained unprocessed in his body. Along with it were all of the emotions that became stuck because he had never let his feelings out. Inside his glass capsule were the details of that experience—the images of those girls standing around him, the feeling of humiliation, the fear of telling anyone, the shame about being so small, and the sound of the kids laughing. He even remembered the pattern of the tile floor in his classroom where the incident happened. Now, still, he panicked whenever there was a situation where he might be in a group or lined up next to others—because it would be obvious how short he was and he was afraid people would notice. All of that energy came rushing back at unexpected times and had been triggering anxiety attacks. In order to help him heal, we needed to go back and work with the elements of the glass capsule to release those details in order to prevent future triggers. We also found other experiences and worked with them, just like you'll be doing in this chapter. But even before that, clearing just that one I shared made a huge difference. You don't have to clear every memory you have; starting with just one or two can help you immensely.

It's important to know that resolving an unprocessed experience from the past is not about forcing yourself to feel happy about it. That's unlikely to happen, which is fine. Resolving it means that you accept that the experience happened and then clear the glass capsule so there is no longer an intense emotional charge or energy disturbance that accompanies it. You don't have to be happy that the experience happened, but you do have to accept that it did and then release that emotional charge we talked about and find a neutrality about it so you can move on.

Identify Unprocessed Experiences to Work With

If your head is spinning and you're wondering how you're supposed to know exactly what experiences from your past are affecting you now, have no fear. I'm going to walk you through that next. In fact, you can relax because you've probably gotten a good head start on clearing some of these unprocessed experiences during your TTT sessions, even though you weren't intentionally aiming for that.

I'm going to show you exactly how to determine what unprocessed experiences might be beneficial to work on. If you don't have any or many memories from your past, don't worry. I'll teach you some tricks for working with experiences of which you have little or no memory.

Use Muscle Testing to Identify Unprocessed Experiences

One very effective way to determine what experiences from your past are still unprocessed and creating anxiety is to tap into your subconscious mind using muscle testing. This is my own go-to method. I love it because you don't have to wrack your brain remembering the experiences from your life and you also won't be swayed by your conscious mind's idea of what seems logical or "big enough" to be tied to anxiety. You just ask your subconscious mind, which already knows the answers and is just waiting to share the information with you. This is also an excellent technique for those who don't remember much from their past. Please don't panic if you aren't comfortable with muscle testing though. I have a great alternative to identifying unprocessed experiences that I'll share next.

With muscle testing, you can use the Standing Test or the O-Ring Test, which you learned in chapter 3. Ask your body out loud or in your head, *Do I have an unprocessed experience contributing to anxiety?*

The answer will almost definitely be "yes." You will probably have many experiences to work on over time, but it takes only one to get started. You can then find out through muscle testing at what age this event occurred, giving you a clue as to what it could be.

Ask, *Did this event occur between the ages of 0–20? 20–30?* and so on. Keep asking until your body answers "yes" to a specific timeline, and then ask about each year within that timeline to get the exact one.

When you've arrived at an age, simply keep an open mind and allow ideas to come to you. Remember, the event could be anything from an obvious experience, like a car accident or an illness, to something you might consider minor. Just be open to whatever comes up.

If you are stuck, ask some additional questions, such as *Is this experience related to a person, my career, my health, etc.?* This process can be quite a guessing game! You are just gathering clues here.

You will keep getting answers from your muscle testing, and eventually you will likely recall the experience or simply have enough information to work with. Even just knowing, for example, that there is an experience from age eight that had something to do with school and your teacher will be enough to clear it.

Once you think you know what the experience is, it's a good idea to double-check it using muscle testing. Remember, your conscious mind may use logic and decide what's linked to what, but the subconscious mind has the original record.

To check your guesswork, ask, *Is the experience (describe it briefly) contributing to anxiety?*

Once you get your confirmation, you will have a tangible experience to work with. Make a note of it so you're ready to go when we get to the clearing technique very soon. If you can't identify or recall the exact experience, just gather as much information about it as you can. For example, through muscle testing you might end up determining that you had an experience at age twenty-four that was linked to your dad, but you can't quite figure out exactly what it was about. No biggie. The body will usually allow us to work with just a few key details if we approach it the right way.

Work with Memories from the Past

Another method of identifying unprocessed experiences is to make a list of memories from your past that you feel you're still holding on to. Jot down the experiences from your life that are still at the forefront of your mind, even if they've long passed.

You're the only one who needs to be able to understand your list, so you can just write things like *the time Mom yelled at me in front of my friend*, *when I fell out of the tree and broke my arm*, or *when our van skidded through the intersection and almost got hit by a truck*. You don't need detailed descriptions.

You may end up with a pretty long list, but that's totally okay. Everyone I know starts with a long list. You can work on this over time. The good news is that you most certainly don't need to clear everything on the list in order to heal from anxiety. Do not judge anything as too small or insignificant to go on the list. Write down everything you can think of.

Here are some questions to jog your memory and help you make your list, plus some examples of possible related events:

- *What still has an emotional charge when you think about it?* Examples: The time so-and-so yelled at me, when I had to move out of the moldy house, when the doctor told me she couldn't do anything for the anxiety.

- *What do you remember that you were "never the same" after?* Examples: A sibling being born, Mom being late to pick you up from school, getting your tonsils out in high school, that time when the boy/girl rejected your invite to the school dance.

- *What experiences can you recall from right before this anxiety showed up in your life?* Examples: A job change, a relationship breakup, an argument with a friend, worrying about a sick parent.

- *What experience still turns your stomach or makes your heart race when you think about it?* Examples: Being left at the lunch table alone in second grade, seeing a car accident on the side of the road, having to put an animal to sleep.

- *What does this anxiety remind you of from the past? Is there a memory you have that triggers emotions similar to what you feel now?* It's very helpful to work on those experiences from the past that remind you of what you are going through now. Examples: When my mom was in the hospital and I didn't know what was going on, when I got fired for something I didn't do, when I was accused of being insensitive to my husband's feelings.

Reminder: If you don't have any or many memories from your past, don't worry. I'm going to show you later on in this chapter how you can still work with unprocessed experiences from your past.

Clear Unprocessed Experiences with EFT

By now you probably have at least a few experiences in mind to work with. If you have a bunch jotted down, that's great, but it can be confusing to know which ones to work with first. As a rule of thumb, choosing any of them by the following means will do:

- If you can muscle-test, simply ask your body, *Would it be most beneficial to clear _____ (describe the experience briefly) first?* Insert any of your experiences in the blank. Keep trying different ones by muscle testing until you get a confirmation of which one to start with.

- Choose the experience that has the greatest emotional charge. What still feels most upsetting? Pick whatever feels biggest.

- Pick an experience intuitively. All of them have a chance of making a big dent in the anxiety, so just pick one and go for it.

- Choose the experience that occurred prior to the onset of the anxiety. I typically tell people to look at what happened about eighteen months to two years before. This won't likely be the only contributing event, but it may be the straw that broke the camel's back, so clearing it could make a huge impact quickly.

You already understand how to use EFT in a simple and effective way for dealing with your feelings in the present moment. But to really clear out the root of anxiety, you need to look at the past and clean out old energies that are likely triggering you. Working with unprocessed experiences is an excellent way to do just that. You'll essentially be opening up that metaphorical glass capsule with all the anxiety-triggering information in it and letting go of it.

Disclaimer: While EFT is easy to use on your own and can be used very safely in the way you first learned it (to deal with your feelings as they arise), I do ask that you tune in to your intuition each time you work with memories from the past (unprocessed experiences) in the way that I'm about to teach you. In the case of very difficult or triggering memories, I encourage you to work with a professional who is trained in this technique. I don't want you to be scared of doing this work on your own, but if something feels very difficult or unsafe for you to think about, it may be too overwhelming for you to clear it on your own. Our bodies are often more secure in the presence of another person who can hold a safe space as we're working through scary emotions, and a professional will have extensive techniques to make sure doing that work is a positive experience for you.

Remember that whether you consider events from your past significant or not, they can still be affecting you in big ways. To address this, we're now going to learn how to use EFT to clear specific memories that are still negatively impacting you (unprocessed experiences).

When using EFT to clear unprocessed experiences from the past, be as specific as you can with the details because it will help clear everything in that glass capsule we learned about earlier.

We'll be using the basic EFT process you already learned and practiced, so the following outline will be very familiar to you. As we go through each step, I'll give you additional directions so you can specifically target and clear unprocessed experiences.

1. Rate the intensity of your experience.

2. Create a set-up statement.

3. Use your set-up statement while tapping the karate chop point.

4. Tap through the rest of the points and vent.

5. Check in and repeat.

6. Wrap up your EFT session.

Step 1: Rate the Intensity of Your Experience

Let's start by clearing whatever memory you identified either by muscle testing or by making your list. Remember, it doesn't matter so much which one you start with, as long as you start. Now give it a simple title or description as a way to reference it for yourself if you haven't already. This might be something like "The day I thought Mom forgot me at school" or "When I had an accident in front of the class in first grade." Close your eyes and recall that memory briefly. Allow the emotions to come to the surface so they are ready to be cleared. On a scale of 1–10, with 10 being the strongest, rate how intense the experience feels for you *now* when you think of it. If you also feel it in your body as a physical sensation, make a mental note of that. If not, no biggie.

Step 2: Create a Set-Up Statement

Based on your experience, create a set-up statement. Just fill in the blanks to modify it for your own situation.

> *Even though _____ (state the experience),*
> *I can be okay anyway.*

You want to use as much descriptive detail as possible to just temporarily bring up the energy of that experience in your system to be cleared. Remember to try to include a physical symptom and emotional feeling in this part of your statement.

Example: *Even though those kids laughed at me when the teacher put me in the corner and I still get a pit in my stomach when I think about it, I can be okay anyway.*

Step 3: Use Your Set-Up Statement While Tapping the Karate Chop Point

Now say the entire set-up statement three times in a row as you tap the karate chop point continuously. Use three or four fingers of one hand to tap the karate chop point of the other hand. Just as I shared in chapter 5 when you learned EFT, you can say the same exact statement three times or change up the words. Once you've completed this step, you are ready to move on to the rest of the tapping points.

Step 4: Tap Through the Rest of the Points and Vent

Next, you are going to simply tap through the rest of the points for several rounds and talk about what happened as you "vent" about the memory. It's best to tell the story and tap in chronological order. For me, it's easiest to tell the story as if I'm talking to a friend, rambling through it all and sharing whatever comes to mind. Just remember to bring up as many details as you can recall while you tap.

If you like your techniques to feel very structured, try the following: Tell the story and tap in segments. You can think of the segments as scenes in a movie. Start at the beginning of the story and tell just the beginning scene or part a few times over as you tap and talk. Continue working with only that scene of the story until you feel emotionally neutral about it when you check in (see step 5). Then you can move on to the next scene and so on.

Whether you tap "Amy style" (like you're blabbing to a friend) or in a more organized way by tapping in segments, pay careful attention to what I call the "sticky" parts of the story—the details that feel most ingrained in your mind or feel most difficult to confront as you tap and vent. You will want to work on those a little bit more in depth.

Lacey was a client of mine who had terrible anxiety around speaking up for herself. Growing up, her mom would often ask Lacey and her sisters what they wanted to eat or wear and then berate them for answering the question the "wrong" way. We both suspected this had contributed to her challenge now. We made a list of her memories and then used muscle testing to identify which unprocessed experience to work with first. When we tapped together, we went through the experience and brought up all the details and feelings about that memory that Lacey could remember.

I gave Lacey the homework of continuing to work with her memories list on her own and reminded her to spend a little extra time on the parts of the memories that felt "sticky" when she recalled them. The sticky parts can be things that simply stand out in your mind or cause the strongest reaction (either physical or emotional) when you talk about them. For Lacey, a few of the sticky details she had to tap through more thoroughly were what her mom's face looked like when Lacey picked out her outfit for the first day of school, the specific color of the dress, and how disappointed Lacey was when her mom threw away that dress after school because Lacey got a tiny marker stain on it.

These types of details might seem little, but if they feel stuck, particularly vivid, or intuitively important for any reason, then really work with them. Doing so will help you process and release your unprocessed experiences in a more complete manner. Focusing on and tapping out the details can make the difference between EFT working so-so and working really well!

Here are some specific ideas of what to include in your tapping:

- *Concrete details of the experience:* Colors, sounds, smells, weather, facial expression, a certain phrase someone said to you that is upsetting, and so on
- *Intangible concepts or feelings:* Feeling used, being unable to trust yourself or someone else, being humiliated, etc.

You're now ready to tap through all of the points from start to finish as you tell your story and vent about whatever comes to mind again. If you're having a hard time telling the story, you can incorporate these general phrases that I often use to help my clients release memories completely:

I'm storing all the details of that experience in my body.

My body is holding on to all the smells, sights, and sounds from that experience.

I still have the details of that experience stuck in my system.

I really remember _____ *(identify a sticky part).*

My body remembers the details of that experience, like

_____.

I remember seeing/hearing/feeling _____.

What we are doing here is prompting the subconscious mind to tap into the details so we can clear them. We "suggest" ideas and triggers to the subconscious mind, and then it works behind the scenes to find those details and clear them.

Step 5: Check In and Repeat

After several rounds of tapping, take a break and check in with yourself. Close your eyes and tune back in to the experience.

Rate the intensity of the experience on a scale of 1–10 again. If you need to keep going, then keep going. (You most likely will.)

Step 6: Wrap Up Your EFT Session

When you have cleared the experience completely or are done with your session until next time, close with a positive round of tapping, from the karate chop point through the rest of the points and back to the karate chop point. You can use *I'm okay* or any other positive statement from chapter 5.

That's it!

Note: Don't forget that Chakra Tapping can be used as an alternative to EFT. Simply use the EFT process I just walked you through, but tap on the chakra points you learned in chapter 5 instead. Other than the set of tapping points you use, everything else is the same: always start with the set-up statement on your karate chop point and go from there.

How Long Should I Tap For?

You should keep tapping until you feel like the memory of your experience is as neutral as it can be. Get your rating as close to 1 as possible! This doesn't have to happen in a single tapping session. So many people make the mistake of tapping for only a couple minutes and then saying, "Tapping doesn't work." While tapping is really effective, it can definitely take time and persistence. Keep working on your memories and feelings, and as you do so, your body will relax more and more because of the burden that is being released.

You will know when the energy attached to the experience has been released from your system when you have a distant or faded vision of your memory. It may feel like it happened to someone else or like it's just "there now" instead of holding a strong emotional charge.

You don't need to completely release each experience before you move on to the next one. I always have a list going of various things I'm working on. I keep going back to them over and over until I feel like they are neutral and I can check them off the list.

If It's Difficult to Recall Specific Experiences

A lot of people come to me panicked when they learn about how important it is to clear experiences from their past. "I don't remember anything!" they tell me. Luckily there is a way around this. You can heal no matter what. Here are some tricks to use if you aren't able to rely on your memory (which is the case for many of us, by the way).

While the ideal way to clear an experience is by tapping and telling the story of your memories in the way I've just taught you, I'm sensitive to the fact that many people don't remember much from their past. If you are one of these people, play around with the following suggestions. These strategies work very well instead of, or as an add-on to, the primary way of clearing an unprocessed experience that you just learned.

Work with Feelings about the Anxiety

Remember, looking at how you feel about the anxiety is a good indicator of what helped to create it. Try to recall times from your past when you felt emotions similar to those you feel now, especially prior to when the anxiety began.

Jim came to me with anxiety and pain in his joints, which had both appeared together about three years prior. I asked him if he remembered what was going on in his life three years ago. He rattled off a list of things that could have caused his body to go into overload. After we explored some initial possibilities, I asked how he felt about the joint pain and anxiety.

Each person will have a unique feeling about their problem, even if the actual problem is a common one such as anxiety. With Jim, I knew that his primary emotion about the joint pain and anxiety would be a good starting point for finding the contributing unprocessed experience. Jim stated that he was "tired of dealing with it [the joint pain and anxiety]." This was the clue we needed in order for him to remember some experiences. I then helped him figure out what else he was "tired of" or what situation had been "tiring" him out during the time period before the symptoms started.

We discovered some marital issues around that time that were making him feel "unworthy." With that, we went to work on clearing energy around specific experiences in his past. That helped immensely not only with Jim's frustration with his situation but also, in time, with his joint pain and anxiety.

Use Mementos from Your Past

Sometimes it's easier to work on a traumatic event from your past by using some reminders to evoke the emotions. This is really helpful when you don't recall the details or are maybe even too detached to "feel" anything about the memory.

Here are some ways to jog your memory:

- Tap while reading past journal entries.
- Write down your story and then tap as you reread it.
- Tell your story to a friend on the phone as you tap.
- Voice-record your experience and then tap along to that.
- Play songs that remind you of that event or time period and tap along. For this one, you don't need to talk, just tap.

Subconscious Tapping

You already know from when you first learned tapping that calling on your subconscious mind during EFT to help is a great way to release old energy, even if you don't know exactly what needs to be cleared. This is a way to work *around* the energy and still work *on* it.

Use this set-up statement: *Even though I have no idea what experiences are causing this anxiety, I give my subconscious permission to release it anyway.* If, through muscle testing, you were able to identify a specific age at which an unprocessed experience occurred but you can't figure out exactly what it was, you could use a set-up statement like this: *Even though I have an unprocessed experience from age ___ that I can't remember, I give my subconscious permission to release it anyway.*

For the rest of the tapping points, focus on the anxiety itself, trying to incorporate any emotions or thoughts you have as you vent.

Tapping through these points might look something like this (saying a different phrase at each point):

> *I don't know what past experiences are making me anxious.*
>
> *Maybe it's _____ (insert any guesses).*
>
> *My subconscious knows exactly what it is.*
>
> *I just can't figure it out like I wish I could.*
>
> *I know that it's from when I was _____ (say the age you were at the time of the experience, if you know it).*
>
> *Subconscious, help me clear this!*

You'll continue tapping through the points in this way for several rounds.

Just keep tapping and talking out loud, which will trigger your subconscious into pulling up whatever it needs to help you clear. This method incorporates a lot of improv, so have fun with it!

The more you practice using EFT, the more ways you'll find to use it. There are no strict rules and there is no need to follow my directions step by step. Really make it your own and I know you'll be pleased with just how effective and versatile this technique can be.

Emotional Freedom Technique (EFT) and Thymus Test and Tap (TTT): A Powerful Combo

While EFT and TTT are two totally different techniques, they complement each other nicely. You can blend the use of these techniques in several different ways. It's all about being creative. Let me share what I did with a client of mine named Linda to give you some ideas.

Linda came to me with a history of lifelong anxiety. She couldn't remember when it started or how, and said it was just "always like this." She did recognize that she felt most anxious when she was alone, which was one clue we worked with. If you write down a brief summary of your challenge, like I just did for Linda's, it might help you dissect it into smaller segments to work with. Here are some of the ways we used EFT and TTT for Linda's challenge. Some of it we did together, and some she did as homework on her own.

- We used TTT over several sessions to release general emotions contributing to anxiety.
- We used TTT to clear emotions triggered when she was alone.

- Using a list of memories from the past when Linda felt alone, we used EFT to clear those experiences.
- We utilized subconscious tapping to clear subconscious causes of anxiety that we may not have picked up with our other approaches.

This process went on for a few weeks until Linda started seeing significant improvement in the anxiety. But we didn't stop there. I had her keep using TTT and EFT, along with clearing harmful beliefs, like you'll be learning in the next chapter. It took about four months for her to get to the point of feeling like anxiety wasn't part of her everyday existence, after suffering for her entire life. As you can imagine, Linda was thrilled with her progress, which ended up requiring less work than she had anticipated.

Summary

Oftentimes entire memories, including all the details of a specific event, get stored in the body and create an imbalance in our system. These unprocessed experiences can become huge triggers for anxiety, being replayed subconsciously without our awareness. They can contribute to constant low-level anxiety or full-blown panic attacks when we least expect them.

Working with unprocessed experiences—past events that we haven't acknowledged, processed, and released—is an amazing way to address the root of anxiety. Using EFT, we can clear details from the figurative glass capsule that's storing various triggers. We do this by talking and tapping at the same time while recalling the stories of past events. We can also explore using TTT and EFT together for a powerful combination.

Chapter Eight

* * * * * * * * * * * * * *

Change Harmful Beliefs

The benefit of changing harmful beliefs can be like striking gold on the path to healing from anxiety! I hope by now you are seeing that there are many ways to clear anxiety. By working with the different techniques that you know, you're slowly addressing the layers of anxiety. Remember, there's no particular order or method to the madness; just keep working on things using what you're learning.

What you're about to learn is going to propel you into a new and exciting world and give you so many opportunities to work toward becoming the most calm, relaxed version of yourself. In this chapter we're going to dive deep into what harmful beliefs are and how to change them using a technique called *The Sweep*, a healing script that I created during my own healing process. I'll also offer specific examples of beliefs that might be affecting you, as a checklist that you can work from.

Discovering these beliefs may shock you, but if you approach the process with curiosity it can actually become quite entertaining. You'll be thinking, *My crazy brain believed what?!* I now consider myself a beliefs detective, and soon you will be one too.

What Beliefs Are

You are probably very familiar with affirmations, which are positive ideas or statements used to create a positive mental shift. But beliefs are ideas that are essentially negative affirmations, working in the opposite way. A belief is simply a message or an idea that you believe to be true. Having a harmful belief is like repeating a negative mantra in your head hundreds of times a day—one your body perceives as truth. Beliefs are based on other people's messages about us, our generalizations about past experiences, and the meanings we make from those experiences. Beliefs are not facts, but to your brain and body, they might as well be. Beliefs are essentially the message you take away from any given experience.

Beliefs are simply messages about things that we believe to be true and are one of the largest causes of anxiety and one of the greatest impediments to overcoming it. The awesome news is that releasing harmful beliefs can be life-changing. Working with and clearing harmful beliefs was perhaps the most important action I took for my own healing and has proven essential to the healing process for my clients, too. I found so many of these beliefs that once I released them, it opened up a path to healing like nothing else I had done. In the same way you unsubscribe to emails that you don't want to keep receiving, you can unsubscribe to your own beliefs. Thank goodness!

Mike grew up in a household with a mother with bipolar disorder. She was particularly unpredictable, often flying off the handle when Mike looked at her in what she described as "the wrong way." Understandably, Mike became very jumpy and anxious when he was home alone with her. Soon he learned that if he stayed in his room and kept quiet, she would leave him alone and not pick fights. The message or belief that Mike intuited from his childhood was "I'm safer when I'm invisible."

This belief directed a lot of his adult behavior, where he always tried to stay out of people's way if they seemed the slightest bit agitated. Mike was often quiet when he wanted to speak up as well. But because he truly believed that he was safer when invisible, he was afraid, which contributed to his anxiety. Working on this belief really helped Mike feel more relaxed around others and be able to voice his thoughts and opinions when he wanted to.

Let's look at a breakdown of the anatomy of a belief and how it affects us:

- Based on our experiences, our subconscious mind perceives a certain message or takeaway from them. (This is the belief.)

- The subconscious creates "rules" that go along with that takeaway. For example, *this* is good or *this* is bad, or when *this* happens then *this* other thing happens.

- These rules become truths that we live by and end up directing our future behavior and feelings.

- We live according to our self-created truths, which create a tainted lens through which we start to see ourselves and our lives, skewing our perceptions.

- We get stuck in a loop where our skewed perspective becomes so ingrained that it keeps us stuck in that belief system, which can cause anxiety.

As you learn about beliefs, the most important thing to remember is not to judge or beat yourself up for having them. We don't create any of this on purpose. It's just part of life! Your job now is not to focus on the past and criticize or analyze it; it's to correct whatever isn't working for you so you can move forward.

The big goal here is to slowly release as many as you can of the subconscious reasons that your body, mind, and spirit are holding on to anxiety. You will probably find a lot of them, and that's okay. Harmful beliefs may be holding you back in big ways, but clearing them is really simple. The cool thing is because beliefs are born from our experiences, you may have inadvertently already knocked out some harmful beliefs while you were releasing stuck energy from the past experiences. What a bonus! We'll do this step by step and one by one.

Examples of the Power of Belief

One of my favorite examples of the power of belief comes from the book, Biology of Belief, written by Bruce Lipton, PhD. Dr. Lipton[6] is an international leader and biologist whose teachings help to bridge the worlds of science and spirit. In the book, he tells the story of a British physician named Dr. Albert Mason. Dr. Mason was using hypnosis to treat a teenage patient's warts. While Dr. Mason had been successful using hypnosis with other patients like this, this particular boy had a very difficult case. His chest was the only place on his body that had normal skin. Their first hypnosis session targeted only on one arm, which improved even after just a week. It was later that a surgeon who had also seen the teenage boy, notified Mason that the issue with his skin was not warts, but in fact, a lethal genetic disease. By using the power of his mind through hypnosis to redirect the boy's subconscious mind into accepting the idea that his skin could and would heal, the impossible occurred—with continued hypnosis sessions, most of the kid's skin became healthy

---

6. Bruce H. Lipton, PhD, *The Biology of Belief: Unleashing the Power of Consciousness, Matter & Miracles* (Carlsbad, CA: Hay House, 2016).

again. There was a huge change in the child's situation because of the transformed belief alone.

What hypnotherapy helped to do in this situation was change only the belief, but nothing else about the circumstances. This is what we're going to be doing with The Sweep. The Sweep is not hypnotherapy, but it works in a similar way wherein it has the ability to reprogram the subconscious mind.

Another example is from the researchers at Victoria University in New Zealand. They managed to trick 148 students into believing they were drunk, even though they had nothing but tonic water and lime. Researchers found that the subjects that believed they were ingesting vodka, had impaired judgment and an actual diminished IQ even though they only believed they had alcohol in their systems.[7]

Two Types of Beliefs

There are two main types of beliefs that each contribute to anxiety in their own way. The category your specific beliefs fall in doesn't matter at all. I just want you to get an idea of how each of these types might be affecting you. Let me explain.

Beliefs That Create Anxiety

The first type of belief is one that actually creates or propels anxiety. These are often beliefs about the world or your life that make you feel unsafe, helpless, and fearful. Beliefs that create anxiety cause you to feel like the world is a scary place, that everyone and everything is out to get you, or that you are totally helpless and unsafe.

Beliefs of this nature constantly make you feel like something is wrong or you are in danger, which triggers your body's

---

7. "Being Drunk 'a Trick of the Mind,'" *BBC News*, January 7, 2003, http://news.bbc.co.uk/2/hi/health/2634499.stm.

fight, flight, or freeze response. While I'll be giving you many examples of specific beliefs later in this chapter, the general idea or message that this type of belief sends is "I am unsafe," which is actually a belief in and of itself. This message can act as that negative affirmation I mentioned before, influencing everything you do, think, and feel. Remember that a belief is simply a message about something, not a truth. Anything you believe that makes you feel unsafe probably triggers anxiety.

Here's an example of how this belief can come into play. When Jimmy was ten years old, he told his parents that he hated his younger sister. While of course this wasn't a nice thing of Jimmy to say, his parents were very upset and put him in timeout for it. They screamed at him and told him never ever to say something like that again. As Jimmy got older, he began to have anxiety, which his parents took him to the doctor for. It almost always got triggered when he was in a situation where he had to share his opinion or feelings. Jimmy's takeaway from what happened with his sister was that sharing his feelings could get him in trouble or make people mad. This became a rule he lived by, which caused him to feel terrified to express how he felt. He ended up with the belief that "when I share my feelings, people get mad at me." This belief not only created anxiety in and of itself but also made it almost impossible for him to comfortably and confidently express his emotions, which then became its own source of anxiety in his life.

Beliefs That Block Healing

The second type of belief is one that actually blocks your healing. This type of belief is one that makes you believe you *need* anxiety for some reason. Even though your conscious mind is doing everything to overcome anxiety, your subconscious mind may be holding what it thinks are very good reasons to have anxiety and *not to heal* from it.

What this means is that at some level, you actually have an inner conflict about letting go of anxiety. This type of inner conflict is very common and happens when one part of us wants to change but the other part (often the subconscious) does not want to change because it believes the change is dangerous or negative for us in some way.

If you have beliefs that are blocking your healing, you may have a pattern of feeling worse the more you do to try to feel better. You may begin to improve but then suddenly slide backward again, or struggle with self-sabotage and find it difficult to help yourself.

The subconscious mind can have programming that makes us believe that anxiety is actually *better* for us than being free from it because it keeps us safe, allows us to do or not do something, and so on. This means that *you* could be the biggest obstacle standing in your own way of overcoming anxiety. This is not your fault, and again, it's very common. There's no reason to be upset about this kind of revelation. Discovering this information is good because it can actually be quite life-changing.

Susan was always afraid of answering questions in front of her class. She was shy from as far back as she could remember and was uncomfortable being the center of attention. In fourth grade though, she was forced to recite a poem at a school assembly. Just before it was her turn, she became dizzy and nauseous. It wasn't until she got older that she was able to identify what she had experienced as a full-blown panic attack. When her teacher saw her crying and obviously not feeling well, she ran over to her and took her to the nurse's office. Susan was relieved that she didn't have to get on that stage. She took that experience and perhaps even subconsciously made the meaning that having an anxiety attack can excuse you from having to do scary things. This became her rule to live by, or a new belief: "I need anxiety to keep me safe." Even though consciously Susan did not want to have anxiety attacks, her subconscious mind knew that this reaction could protect her, and it became her body's default response to having to be the center of attention.

In both of these examples, the way an elementary-school child saw the world stayed with that child into adulthood. This doesn't happen with every experience you have, so you don't need to worry that you'll have to undo everything you've ever learned. And it's no one's fault that these beliefs get formed, so please don't be angry with your parents and teachers for every belief you find. Beliefs are just part of being human. You just need to address the messages or beliefs that aren't working for you anymore. Healing from anxiety is in part about unlearning or unbelieving anything that is blocking you from being calm and relaxed. The way your seven-year-old self saw things may have been okay when you were seven, but unless you would allow a seven-year-old to run your life now (can you imagine?!), it's definitely time to update your mental records.

Identify Your Beliefs

Now we're on to the really important stuff—figuring out what beliefs are actually affecting you. I'll remind you again that there may be a ton of beliefs to work on. We're talking mountains and mountains of them. But don't worry, you don't need to rush and you won't have to release every last one in order to heal. You just need to make a good dent in the pile. Clearing even one belief can make a huge difference in your life.

Typically, beliefs are built around a few main concepts:

Safety (*It's unsafe to heal*)—If part of us doesn't feel *safe* to heal from anxiety, it can block every effort we make to overcome it. This is the block I see most often, even though it seems so illogical, as anxiety is typically associated with making us feel unsafe. But there are many ways it can protect us, too.

Deserving (*I'm undeserving of healing*)—This block is so common and is all about not believing that we truly deserve to be healthy and happy. This has to do with self-worth and not feeling good enough.

Ability (*I'm unable to heal no matter what*)—This block is linked to all the reasons that we believe we aren't able to heal, such as not having enough money, energy, resources, etc.

Willingness (*I'm unwilling to heal*)—This is related to the idea that we aren't willing to do what it takes to heal, energy-wise, financially, or otherwise. This block primarily has to do with the "work" involved in healing. This belief is not based in laziness but often comes from being drained of gusto after a long dance with our challenge.

Readiness (*I'm not ready to heal*)—Not feeling ready to heal can play a part when we feel like things would change too fast or there is more we need to do before we'll be ready to get back to life.

Possibility (*It's impossible to heal*)—The feeling that it's not possible to heal often comes from the medical professionals who are trying to help us. Hearing that we have the "most severe case" of something or that our issue is "incurable" gives ammunition to these types of beliefs. This block is built around feeling like our circumstances are just too bad for us to heal.

Wanting (*I don't want to heal*)—Not wanting to heal usually comes from having an upside to our challenge. Everything that we perceive as negative in our lives (such as illness) also has a positive aspect (a benefit). Sometimes, even if only at a subconscious level, the benefit we gain from the challenge prevents us from wanting to overcome it.

A List of Common Beliefs

This list of common harmful beliefs that can block healing covers many of the main concepts I just laid out. It is meant to be a starting point to help you brainstorm. For now, I want you to get a good sense of just how many silly ideas your brain might have, so you'll be really excited about the clearing you'll get to do soon. The following list will open your eyes to the possibilities of crazy beliefs that could be keeping you stuck. If you want, you can put a star or check by beliefs you may want to work with later. Remember that these beliefs could be either those that are *creating anxiety* (essentially causing you stress in some way) or those that are *blocking you from healing* (making part of you feel that having anxiety is *better* for some reason than healing from it), or even a mix of both.

With the list of beliefs, it's best to tailor the wording to your specific situation as much as possible. For instance, some of the beliefs I've suggested are fairly general, such as "I need anxiety." If you can add a "because…" and elaborate just a bit (example: "because it's the only way I can say no"), it will be even more powerful for your healing.

- *I need anxiety.*
- *The world is unsafe.*
- *I'm not good enough.*
- *I am undeserving of health and happiness.*
- *People will hate me if I share my opinions/feelings.*

- *I'll be ridiculed if I _____.*
- *No one loves me.*
- *Everything is my fault.*
- *I'm too sensitive to be out in the world.*
- *I'm broken.*
- *I'm unlovable.*
- *I always make the wrong decision.*
- *When things start to go well, something bad happens.*
- *If I do what I want, other people will be unhappy.*
- *Being healthy and happy at the same time is impossible.*
- *I'll only be loved if I'm perfect.*
- *I have to hold all of my emotions in.*
- *If I do something good for myself, someone else will be upset.*
- *Anxiety is my punishment for doing something bad in the past.*
- *Having anxiety is my only legitimate excuse to stay home.*
- *Having anxiety is the only way I can say no.*
- *Anxiety allows me not to be social.*
- *I'll only be loved/taken care of if I have anxiety.*
- *I need anxiety to feel safe because _____.*
- *It's unsafe to express my emotions.*
- *It's unsafe to be my true self.*
- *I'm undeserving of relaxation.*
- *I deserve anxiety because of something I did in the past.*
- *I'm undeserving of love.*
- *I don't matter.*
- *I'm worthless.*

- *Nothing will work for me.*
- *Everyone else can heal, but I can't.*
- *Overcoming anxiety is impossible.*
- *Overcoming anxiety will take too much work.*
- *I need this anxiety to have my needs met.*
- *If I heal, it will just come back.*
- *I'll end up alone if I heal. (People only stick around because I have anxiety.)*
- *It's unsafe to relax.*
- *It's unsafe to be happy.*
- *I'll want to leave my relationship if I heal.*
- *I can only heal with more support.*
- *I'm only worthy when _____ (I'm perfect, I'm doing things for others, etc.).*
- *I can only heal with more money.*
- *If I get well and still can't find a partner, I'll have no excuse.*
- *Healing would prove this was my fault in the first place.*
- *I will be too vulnerable if I heal.*
- *I'll have nothing to do if I heal.*
- *There's no point to healing. (I have no purpose worth healing for.)*
- *I have to forgive others in order to heal and then they'll be off the hook.*
- *I will lose my identity if I heal.*
- *I'm too far behind in life to ever catch up.*
- *I have to live up to others' (or my own) expectations.*
- *I have to be perfect.*

- *I'm going to let myself down.*
- *I don't know how to heal.*
- *I'll have to be more assertive if I heal.*
- *I'm not strong enough to heal.*
- *I don't have what it takes to heal.*
- *I'm too sensitive to heal.*
- *I'm too delicate to heal.*
- *I'm delicate and/or I'm sensitive.*
- *I'm unable to handle life.*
- *I need this anxiety as a distraction (from my unhappy life, my marriage, my job, etc.).*
- *It will be unfair to the other people who are still suffering if I heal.*
- *My life will change if I heal (and that's too scary).*
- *I'll hurt my doctor's/friends'/family's feelings if I don't heal their way.*
- *I'll have to be successful if I heal.*
- *I'll have to leave an unhealthy relationship if I heal.*
- *It's too much work and I don't have the energy left to heal.*
- *I'll lose my financial benefits if I heal.*
- *I might lose my support system if I heal.*
- *Nothing will work anyway.*
- *People will only believe I'm in pain if they see me suffering.*
- *I've always had this problem and I always will.*
- *Everyone else is smarter than me, so it's easier for them.*
- *I'm too damaged to heal.*
- *Someone has to suffer, and maybe it's meant to be me.*

- *I can only grow spiritually when I'm suffering.*
- *Getting better will change my relationship with someone I love.*
- *My life will be too stressful if I'm healthy.*
- *I'll have to be social if I heal.*
- *I won't have an excuse if I fail or quit something if I heal.*
- *I will have to live up to my full potential if I heal.*
- *No one will take care of me if I heal.*
- *I will need to figure out my life if I heal.*
- *I will have to be intimate with my spouse if I heal.*
- *I'll have to be present for my children if I heal.*

Are you starting to see that nothing is off limits as far as beliefs go? Good. That's going to help you big time during this process.

Optional: Muscle-Test to Identify and Confirm Beliefs

While not necessary, if you want to confirm if certain beliefs are contributing to anxiety for you, make use of muscle testing. Simply state a belief from the previous list and test. Remember, your body will tell you what's true for you. If that belief isn't working for you, it's something that needs to be released or shifted, which we'll be doing shortly.

Muscle testing for a belief might go something like this:

Say out loud, *Everyone else can do it, but I can't.*

If your body leans forward using the Standing Test or your fingers stay strong during the O-Ring Test, that means it's true for you. If your body leans backward during the Standing Test or your fingers weaken during the O-Ring Test, then your body is saying it's not true for you, and you can move on to the next belief and test. Please note that it will never hurt to clear a belief "just in case." So if you aren't able to muscle-test for it but think it could apply to you, clear it to be on the safe side.

You only need to choose one belief to start the clearing process. You can go back and work on the rest later. Again, there's no need to try to create some organized system for "getting them all." Follow your intuition and clear the beliefs as they come to you (but write them down in case they come at you faster than you can clear them).

Use The Sweep Technique to Clear Beliefs

The Sweep is a super simple technique that clears beliefs by gently sweeping them out of the subconscious mind.

As you know, the subconscious mind's programming can be pretty stubborn. What's stuck in there is the result of many things that have convinced you to believe certain ideas. The great thing is that the subconscious and conscious minds are designed to work together, like a buddy system. That allows us to fully utilize our conscious mind (the part of us that knowingly really wants to heal) and gently influence our subconscious mind to let go of old beliefs, perceptions, and more.

The Sweep lets us reprogram the subconscious mind through a very simple conversational script. We're going to use the specific verbiage that I've created to do this. The Sweep is *not* hypnosis, but it does relax the body and brain enough to allow us to change their programming. For this reason, some people get really relaxed or feel a bit zoned-out while using The Sweep. You will be in total control though the entire time.

I included the phrase *I am now free…* in almost every sentence of The Sweep. This phrase is a key to the entire process. Freedom is a natural human desire, and it is counterintuitive for a human being to resist it in any way. Even the stubborn subconscious mind won't push that one away.

I suggest that you record this verbiage on your phone so you can fully relax as you listen and repeat along. With this technique, you may notice that your mind wanders. Just let it do so, as there are two reasons for this. It might be a sign that there are energies associated with those thoughts that are trying to clear, or it might indicate that you're in a deep state of reprogramming that bypasses your conscious mind, so it's free to think or wander.

Yawning, sighing, getting the chills, feeling emotional, burping, stomach gurgling and other signals along these lines are good indicators of energy moving. You may also feel nothing at all, which is fine.

The Sweep ticks the boxes for what is needed to successfully reprogram these beliefs:

Acknowledge. We need to acknowledge that we have this belief and that it's not working for us anymore. You've probably noticed a pattern by now—a simple acknowledgment of your emotions, beliefs, and patterns is a big part of letting them go.

Trust. Like us, the subconscious mind responds more positively when we treat it with kindness and compassion, as we would a friend. We need the subconscious mind on our side for this to work. That means it has to feel safe enough to relax and agree to release old beliefs.

Replace. This means we need to replace the old harmful belief with a new and healthier belief. The last part of The Sweep allows us to install a positive belief to go forward with. It's pretty cool that we get to choose something we'd rather believe and give it to the subconscious mind as a better option.

The Sweep Script

Begin by placing your hands over your heart to connect with your inner being or higher self. Now simply repeat the script slowly and deliberately, taking a breath in between each phrase or line. Don't rush through the process, as it's most effective to go slowly when working with the subconscious mind.

Even though I have this belief _____ (state the belief), I acknowledge it's no longer working for me.

I am now free to thank it for serving me in the past, when maybe I really needed it.

I am now free to release all resistance to letting it go.

I am now free to release all ideas that I need this to stay safe.

I am now free to release all ideas that I need it for any reason.

I am now free to release all feelings that I don't deserve to let it go.

I am now free to release all conscious and subconscious causes of it.

I am now free to release all patterns, emotions, and memories connected to it.

I am now free to release all generational or past-life energies keeping it stuck.

All of my being is healing and clearing this energy now, including any stress responses stored in my cells.

Healing, healing, healing.
Clearing, clearing, clearing.

It is now time to install the belief of _____ (Insert a
positive belief here. It can be the opposite of the belief you
are releasing or simply a general positive statement, such
as "I can be calm and free.").

Installing, installing, installing.

And so it is done.

When you're finished, take a few deep breaths. I suggest that you repeat the script a few times in a row (start with two). If you use muscle testing, confirm that you cleared the belief completely by stating it out loud again, and see if your body still resonates or agrees with it. If it does, keep using The Sweep. If it's no longer true for you, then yay! You're done!

If for some reason the belief didn't clear completely, don't worry at all. You can just repeat The Sweep again and retest. This process can take a few rounds of slow, deliberate intention and focus.

Tip: The Sweep can also be used effectively for clearing layers of energy contributing to anxiety. Instead of inserting a belief into the verbiage, you might use something like this: *Even though I have this _____ (anxiety, fear of being alone, racing heart, etc.), I acknowledge that it's no longer working for me.* Then revise the wording to fit your specific focus and repeat a few times.

Additional Ways to Clear Beliefs

While The Sweep is an easy and effective way to clear beliefs, you are probably starting to see that there are many ways to work with each aspect of your healing. Here are some additional ways to work with beliefs that I find very powerful. Feel free to combine techniques, like I tend to do, or just pick your favorite and stick with that one.

Use Tapping for the Belief

In my work with clients and myself, I often work on clearing beliefs using EFT or Chakra Tapping too. It's simple! You can do this instead of The Sweep or as another layer to addressing them. To use tapping for clearing beliefs, simply create the set-up statement and state the belief in the fill-in-the-blank portion (while tapping on the karate chop point). Then, when you tap through the rest of the points and vent, talk about that belief (how it makes you feel, where you might have gotten it, and more). You can also state the belief out loud as you tap if you're having trouble figuring out what to talk about. When using tapping to clear beliefs, you are essentially using the same process as when you work with unprocessed experiences, but you are focusing on a belief instead of an experience.

Find a Connected Unprocessed Experience

With most beliefs, the only requirement to clear them from our body is to simply acknowledge the belief itself. For other beliefs, we may benefit from clearing energy connected to the origin point of the belief—likely an unprocessed experience from the past. Remember, our interpretations of past experiences are where we get messages that then become the beliefs (rules) that we live by.

The best way to know if clearing a related unprocessed experience is necessary, and that's through muscle testing. If you haven't quite mastered muscle testing yet, don't worry. I'm going to give you an alternative way to work with unprocessed experiences connected to your beliefs.

Here's what to ask using muscle testing: *Would it be beneficial to clear an unprocessed experience that helped create the belief that _____ (state the belief)?*

If you get a "yes," your body is saying there is more energy that would be beneficial to clear. At this point you can go back to chapter 7, where you learned about identifying and clearing unprocessed experiences. Use the method of finding unprocessed experiences, but alter the muscle-testing question to refer to the belief you're working with. You might ask something like this: *Is this belief linked to an experience from between the ages of 0–20?* And so on, until you identify the age and the experience. You are essentially going back to figure out where your body got the idea that this belief was true.

If you're still working on mastering the art of muscle testing and aren't confident in it yet, you can find a related experience anyway. Do this by thinking about past experiences that might be connected to the belief you want to clear. You can ask yourself the question *Is there an experience from my past that could have helped send me the message of that belief?* Usually something will pop up. Then you'll clear that in the same way you would any unprocessed experience.

Use Thymus Test and Tap (TTT)

Because beliefs come from experiences, and stuck emotions are often connected to experiences as well, here's a little trick: Use TTT to clear emotions related to the belief you are working on. Using muscle testing and the list of unprocessed emotions from chapter 6, simply ask your body, *Can I find and release a stuck emotion linked to the belief that _____ (state the belief)?* You can also use the other method of identifying emotions from chapter 6, which is swirling your finger over the list.

Working with an unprocessed experience linked to a belief is not an absolutely necessary step, but it can help clear the energy behind the belief more completely for better results.

How Emotions, Experiences, and Beliefs Are Connected

Now you have a good understanding of how stuck emotions and unprocessed experiences affect you (from chapters 6 and 7). You also see how beliefs can both cause anxiety and block you from healing. To tie this all together, let me show you how strongly all of this is connected and why working on all of these aspects during your healing journey can be so transformational. I want to remind you here again that there is no totally perfect or organized way of doing this. The process is all about working on whatever you can think of to work on, and knowing that most of it is more interconnected than you might think. There's not necessarily a streamlined, step-by-step way or order in which to do this, although you will be able to use the guide to anxiety-healing protocols in chapter 9 to get some ideas to follow for your clearing.

Sandy was new to energy work and came to me with anxiety that she described as "always feeling shaky on the inside." She had grown up with an alcoholic father and told me that she had always been on edge in the morning because that's when he was most stressed. Because he was unable to drink in the morning since he had to go to work, his frustration caused him to lash out at family members.

Sandy had never been relaxed in her home while growing up. She had always made sure she was on her best behavior, not calling any attention to herself. Now, even at fifty years old, she was never relaxed. This meant that her nervous system was always frazzled and she was living in fight, flight, or freeze mode.

She always felt on edge, especially in the morning. I have heard different versions of this story from many, many clients, and I think most of us can relate to it in some way, even if we didn't grow up with an alcoholic parent. Growing up with instability—an ill parent, a parent who was out of work, etc.—can cause a very similar reaction.

First, I taught Sandy about the fight, flight, or freeze response and how her nervous system would benefit greatly from some retraining, which you learned in chapter 4. She began doing those exercises daily.

Sandy's body was still storing stuck emotions, which caused her to feel those emotions all the time, triggering her fight, flight, or freeze response almost constantly. Mornings were the most anxiety-filled for her, as her body was still holding the emotional energy associated with that time of day. The body is so smart!

Sandy and I started by doing some work using the techniques you learned in previous chapters. We used TTT to release emotions linked to her father, to the mornings, and to feeling unsafe. We also used EFT to work on a few experiences from the past that stood out strongly in her mind, particularly scary mornings. But she had some harmful beliefs, or rules, that she was living by that we needed to address too.

The first harmful belief that we discovered and cleared was "I am unsafe in the mornings." That was true for Sandy when she was young, and she still believed it as a grown woman. The second belief was "If I'm perfect, things will be okay." Again, that was true for her when she was little because if she didn't make noise or waves, her dad would ignore her. However, it's impossible to be perfect, so any perceived mess-up on her part as an adult would throw her into an anxiety tailspin, causing her to believe something bad would happen.

On top of that, Sandy resonated with the belief that "anxiety keeps me safe." Because she had been so anxious around her dad, she had been hyperaware of her actions and could prevent herself from getting picked on by him. The belief that "anxiety keeps me safe" is probably the most common one I see. This always surprises clients because anxiety tends to make us feel unsafe, at least consciously.

These beliefs I just described were both creating anxiety for Sandy *and* blocking her from healing from it. She emailed me a couple weeks later in shock that those beliefs had been keeping her so stuck. She said that she had never felt as good as she did since releasing them. I suspect that the beliefs we cleared were just the straw that broke the camel's back, so to speak. All of the stuck emotions and unprocessed experiences she cleared were also very important. Again, the discoveries we make don't have to be huge, but the weight of releasing them one by one, as they are revealed to us, can be everything.

At first it may seem overwhelming to figure out what beliefs you're living by, but you're pretty much reciting your beliefs in your head all day long! "I'll never be successful." "This anxiety is going to ruin my life." "I have to be perfect or Mom won't love me." And Sandy and I could have been successful even if we had worked with a different set of beliefs. As long as you are releasing old emotional energy, you are making progress!

In order to engage your brain in thinking about beliefs related to specific unprocessed experiences, ask yourself, "What message did I take away from that experience, or what might I now believe because of it?" Don't forget, you have the mega list of beliefs that I provided earlier in this chapter to work with too.

Summary

Beliefs are not facts, but instead are simply how we see things based on our experiences and our interpretations of them. Much of the information about our lives resides in the subconscious mind and dictates our behavior and our reality.

Beliefs can both create anxiety *and* block us from healing from it. The tough part is that you might not have been aware that this was going on. But now that you do, you can change it.

Using The Sweep technique is a very effective way to transform these beliefs. In addition to working with the belief itself, it's always helpful to release any stuck emotions and clear any unprocessed experiences that you think could be related to it. By using this approach, you are working not only with the belief but also with other energies that contributed to that belief in the first place, which leads to the deepest clearing possible.

Section IV

* * * * * * * * * * * * * * * *

Putting It All Together

Chapter Nine

✳ ✳ ✳ ✳ ✳ ✳ ✳ ✳ ✳ ✳ ✳ ✳ ✳ ✳ ✳

Guide to
Anxiety-Healing Protocols

By now, you know so much about the energetic approach to healing anxiety. In this chapter let's tie everything you've learned together so you can see it all at a glance.

Remember, healing from anxiety comes from focusing on these five things:

- Calm and retrain your body

- Deal with your feelings

- Release stuck emotions

- Release unprocessed experiences from the past

- Change harmful beliefs

As long as you are slowly chipping away at addressing them, little by little, you are healing anxiety. It's your job to keep working with those techniques until you reach the ultimate big-picture finish line of a relaxed and happy you.

In this chapter, we'll review all the tools and processes you already know from previous chapters. I'll also give you plenty of concrete ideas on how to use them.

As I keep reminding you, there's no need to go in any specific order of what energies to address for healing anxiety. Simply hit the ground running and work with whatever issues you're led to explore. You can muscle-test to see what's best to start working with, jump around from thing to thing, or just start somewhere. It all works!

Sample Anxiety Healing Protocols

Here are some general starting-point protocols so you can easily see how you can take everything you've learned and use it together. These protocols are ones I built quickly taking different pieces of what you know and blending them for you. Feel free to expand on and revise any of these protocols to meet your needs.

Sample Protocol A

- Muscle-test to see if your body believes you need anxiety. If you get a "yes," ask yourself why that might be true. Clear *I need anxiety because* _____ using The Sweep a few times. If you have multiple beliefs along the lines of needing anxiety, clear each one. You can use EFT or Chakra Tapping rather than The Sweep if you prefer.

- Use EFT or Chakra Tapping to work on how you feel about the anxiety.

- See if you can think of an experience from your past where you felt the same way that you do now about the anxiety. For example, if you are sad that you are experiencing anxiety, what other time in your life pops into your head about when you were sad? Use EFT to clear the experience, as the two may likely be connected in some way.

- Think about what happened just before the anxiety started (usually up to two years prior). Use EFT or Chakra Tapping for those experiences.

- Use TTT to release *emotions contributing to anxiety.* Repeat for several sessions.

- Clear a few beliefs such as "I'm unsafe in the world" and "I'm undeserving of health and happiness." Look at the list I provided in chapter 8 and continue working on beliefs. You can use The Sweep or EFT/Chakra Tapping for this.

Sample Protocol B

- Clear the belief that *I have to suppress my emotions* using The Sweep a few times. You can use EFT or Chakra Tapping rather than The Sweep, if you prefer.

- Use TTT to release *emotions triggering the fight, flight, or freeze response.* Repeat over several sessions.

- Is there a certain experience you feel like you've never let go of from your past, especially before the onset of anxiety? Use EFT/Chakra Tapping to release it.

- Use subconscious tapping to clear the energy of anxiety. Repeat over several sessions or even daily.

- Think about how anxiety serves you. Are you afraid in any way to let go of it? For example, does it help you say no to things you'd otherwise feel pressured to say yes to? Use EFT to tap about how it serves you so you can release that energy.

Directory of Techniques and Ways to Use Them

Here is a quick directory of techniques you can use to heal anxiety, including when and how to use them and where in the book to find them.

Techniques to Calm the Fight, Flight, or Freeze Response

Chapter 4: Calm and Retrain Your Body

The techniques you learned in chapter 4 are essential for getting your body out of flight, fight, or freeze mode (aka freak-out mode) and into healing mode. Doing these techniques daily and with consistency is key.

Here are some other wonderful ways to apply the calming and retraining techniques from that chapter:

- Use them when you are feeling too scattered to focus on energy work.

- Apply them in the moment if you are panicked or feeling intense emotion.

- Utilize them as a go-to tool for resetting and grounding your energy, much like you'd use deep breathing or meditation.

- Practice them prior to using other techniques in order to help your clearing go more smoothly.

- Do them before you go into a crowd or are around people who trigger you as a way to strengthen and protect your energy.

Thymus Test and Tap (TTT)

Chapter 6: Release Stuck Emotions

Use TTT to release emotions in the following categories. Remember, there may be lots and lots of emotions in your body. Each person can have thousands, but you don't need to clear even close to all of them in order to see improvement. Using TTT can produce almost instant results, but working with it long term should be seen as a marathon and not a sprint. Simply go to the list of unprocessed emotions in chapter 6 (page 120) and ask via muscle testing, *Can I find and release an emotion that is …*

- *contributing to anxiety?*
- *making it difficult for me to heal from anxiety?*
- *related to a specific age in my life?* (If you get a "yes," you will need to muscle-test to identify the age or choose an age.)
- *related to a specific experience from my past?* (If you get a "yes," you will need to muscle-test to identify the age and figure out what happened at that time.)
- *triggered by a specific person in my life?* (If you get a "yes," you will need to muscle-test to identify the person or choose a person to work on clearing energy around.) Please note that this is not a pass to blame anyone. A person can be triggering old energy from the past, even from something that happened long before you met them.
- *linked to a specific place?* (If you get a "yes," you will need to muscle-test to identify the place or choose a place to work with. For example, it could be a childhood home, a place of employment, a specific city, etc.)

Note: If you are unable to muscle-test for any reason, use the other method described in that section of swirling your finger around the list to identify the specific emotions you need to release. (See option B on page 122.)

Emotional Freedom Technique (EFT) and Chakra Tapping
Chapter 5: Deal With Your Feelings

EFT and Chakra Tapping are both excellent techniques to help you process and release old energy from your body. You can use tapping in the following ways:

- For how you feel in any given moment (Tapping is a wonderful way to release stress, tension, and anxiety as it comes up.)

- To work with how you feel *about* anxiety (for example, frustrated, disgusted, grief-stricken, etc.)

- To release unprocessed experiences from your past

- To clear beliefs (as an alternative or in addition to using The Sweep)

The Sweep

Chapter 8: Change Harmful Beliefs

The Sweep is a gentle yet powerful tapping script that helps you use the partnership between your conscious and subconscious minds to release old energy. With this technique, you gently usher out energies that no longer serve you and install something positive. You can fill in the blank at the beginning of the script with anything you want to release, such as the following:

- A belief

- Specific fears

- Energy related to a specific person, place, or thing (for example, *energy related to work, to my childhood home, to elevators, etc.*)

- Any general statement related to anxiety (such as *the causes of anxiety*)

- A specific problem (like *anxiety*)

- A physical symptom of anxiety (for example, *this racing heart*)

Use Muscle Testing to Choose a Technique

Once you're comfortable with all of the techniques in the book, it's fun to use muscle testing to determine which ones would be most beneficial for you to use depending on what you're working on. As you've seen in this chapter, there are many ways to use each technique. You can certainly just choose whatever technique you want to work with, but you can also use muscle testing to tap into your body's wisdom.

Simply ask the question *Would it be most beneficial to clear* _____ *(insert a short description of whatever you're clearing, such as "the belief that I'm not good enough") using* _____ *(insert the name of any technique)?* Depending on what technique your body says yes to, you can then create a plan for how to address the issue. Alternatively, you can write all the techniques you're considering using on a piece of paper. Then use the technique where you swirl your finger around the page to see what technique you're drawn to.

It's important to know that it's common to have to layer techniques (use more than one) in order to clear a specific issue completely. For example, your body may want to clear the belief that "I'm not good enough" first by using The Sweep (you can even muscle-test to see how many times you need to do it) and then by following up with a few minutes of EFT. Be creative and open-minded! The more curious you are, the easier working on healing becomes.

Ways to Address the Root of Anxiety

We've talked a lot about the different energies we need to address to work with the root of anxiety: releasing stuck emotions, clearing unprocessed experiences, and changing harmful beliefs. Here are some specific ideas for exactly how to apply the techniques to each of those types of energies.

Stuck Emotions

Chapter 6: Release Stuck Emotions

Working to release stuck emotions with TTT is one of my favorite ways to start making a dent in clearing an issue! Here are some ideas of what to focus on when clearing stuck emotions. You can address whatever you feel applies to you, or ask with muscle testing, *Can I release an emotion linked to…*

- Energy in a specific part of the body (It's helpful to address the area where you feel the symptoms of anxiety, if any.)
- A specific person (*Mom, Dad, etc.*)
- A time period in your life (*high school, my first job, etc.*)
- A specific job (*when I worked at _____*)
- A theme (such as *intimate relationships* or *difficulty finding jobs*)
- A fear you have (such as *a fear of flying*)
- A pattern that's hard for you to break (*self-sabotage, being critical, etc.*)
- A specific place (such as *my childhood home*)
- A symptom (*digestive issues, migraines, etc.*)
- A specific age (*age 10, age 37, etc.*)

Unprocessed Experiences

Chapter 7: Clear Unprocessed Experiences

The unprocessed experiences from your past will likely be plentiful! Clearing them can make a big difference, even if you don't recall every detail of an experience or aren't sure if it was a big deal anyway.

- Identify beliefs to clear either by jogging your memory or muscle testing. You may have a lot of them, but having a running list of beliefs to work on over time is great!

- Clear the experiences using EFT and/or Chakra Tapping.

- Release stuck emotions related to those specific experiences using TTT. Ask via muscle testing, *Can I clear a stuck emotion from _____ (state the experience)?* Or use the alternative method of swirling your finger around the list of unprocessed emotions (on page 120) to identify which emotions to clear.

Harmful Beliefs

Chapter 8: Change Harmful Beliefs

Almost everyone who has experienced anxiety for a period of time has some reason (often subconscious) for holding on to it. We often find those reasons rooted in our hidden beliefs. Here are some very effective ways to identify and change harmful beliefs:

- Make a list of stressful messages you have about yourself and the world that might be causing anxiety. Some examples: *Everyone is out to get me, Life's not fair, There's never enough money,* and so on.

- Make a list of reasons why your subconscious mind might believe you need anxiety. Ask this powerful question: *If my brain had some crazy idea of why I shouldn't heal, what would it be?*

- If you're able, use muscle testing to confirm which beliefs are true for you at a core level. (If you can't confirm, clear them anyway to be safe.)

- Clear the beliefs you've identified using The Sweep. Fill in the first blank with the belief you wish to clear.

- Use EFT or Chakra Tapping to clear specific unprocessed experiences from the past that gave you the message you need anxiety.

- Try to think of experiences from the past where anxiety was a benefit in some way (for example, it gave you an excuse to take care of yourself). Clear these experiences using EFT or Chakra Tapping.

- Use TTT to clear emotions that are causing you to hold on to anxiety.

Now you have some great guidelines for clearing anxiety that you can refer back to over and over again. These are the exact same approaches that thousands of others have used for their healing. Now it's your turn. Remember to incorporate any ideas you have as they come up and really make this your own.

Ryan's Story: An In-Depth Healing Example

The best way to learn is to read about a real-life example of how anxiety can be addressed by integrating all that you've learned. Through Ryan's story, I'm going to show you how I approached his particular situation. My intention in sharing the specifics of what Ryan and I worked on and how we did it is to give you the support, ideas, and permission you need to think like a detective and feel confident working on clearing your own emotional baggage. Writing out your own story on paper might help you more easily identify the layers you could work with for yourself.

Note that the way I dissect Ryan's story and address each part may be totally different from how you'd do it, and we would both be "right." There are so many different ways to address anxiety that any combination can result in great improvement.

Ryan came to me for help because his whole life was consumed by anxiety. In fact, as I see often, it was affecting his physical body too. He had been diagnosed with irritable bowel syndrome and had lower back spasms. When he first began experiencing anxiety, everything would tighten up when he became anxious and he would feel so out of control. But by the time I met him, he was pretty much in a constant state of emotional and physical distress. He had been seeing various doctors, psychotherapists, and hypnotherapists for five years by the time we began working together. I encouraged him to continue doing what he was already doing, but to add in my approach of addressing emotional baggage.

Action Item: I immediately started Ryan on a schedule of calming and retraining his body, just as you learned to do in chapter 4. His goal was to practice the exercises three times a day, for a few minutes each.

After teaching Ryan the Standing Test, we first asked Ryan's body through muscle testing if it believed that he needed the anxiety. This is one of the first questions I explore with clients, because it provides an easy explanation for why things are stuck. I'm basically testing to see if the body sees anxiety as beneficial or useful in some way, which is very common. I knew that if that *need* resonated with his body, it could take some time to figure out all the reasons why he might believe that (but it would be well worth our time). We got a "yes" response. At a deep subconscious level, Ryan did believe that he needed anxiety. Together, we came up with a list of beliefs, or reasons, his body might have for not wanting to let go of the anxiety.

Safety is one of the primary reasons the body holds on to anxiety. So we asked his body in the first person, *Do I need the anxiety to help me stay safe?* Ryan's body signaled a "yes." Ryan was a little surprised, but he was a great sport! We kept exploring.

While it wasn't necessary, we asked Ryan's body through muscle testing, *Does anxiety keep me safe emotionally?* (Some other options would be *financially* or *physically*.) Again, the answer was a "yes." We could have just left the belief as "Anxiety keeps me safe," but finding out *why*, if possible, always helps us clear it more completely. We talked about this for a little bit, and at first Ryan described this answer as "crazy," because anxiety actually made him feel *unsafe*. But the more we discussed it, the more he could see it being a possibility. He said, "Having anxiety keeps me from having to really be out there in the world. I guess I can kind of lay low and have an excuse." Aha! That totally made sense. Ryan said that for his whole life he had always put so much pressure on himself financially and socially, especially after he graduated from college.

Action Item: Ryan had the belief that "anxiety keeps me safe because it prevents me from having to be out in the world." We used The Sweep technique and repeated it four times until we used muscle testing to confirm that the energy attached to this belief was completely gone.

We could have easily just cleared the belief itself to see if that would help. But because I usually try to dig deeper into every clue I find, I wondered where this energy originated.

That's when we started testing ages to find out when this need for anxiety actually originated so we could see if there were any other energies to clear from that time. I typically break the age ranges down into twenty-year periods (ages 0–20, 20–40, etc.) and test for each. I knew Ryan's body had the recording of exactly when this energy imbalance that triggered the anxiety started in his system.

Is this belief that anxiety keeps me safe linked to an age between 0–20? His body let us know the answer was "no." *Is it linked to ages 20–40?* We got a "yes" and then narrowed it down to the exact age by breaking it down to ten years, five years, and then individual years. His body told us through muscle testing that the itching was linked to age 22. Because we now had another clue to what was connected to the anxiety, it was another energy we could clear. Hooray!

Action Item: We used TTT to release about thirty stuck emotions from age 22.

Ryan and I chatted about what was going on that year and came up with a few solid things. We weren't focused on looking for traumatic events from his past, because we had already talked about how pretty much *anything* could be the culprit, even if it seemed like no big deal. Instead, we just discussed what was going on in general during that time period. Ryan had just graduated from college and was looking for a job. He found the company of his dreams, and then after three rounds of interviews, he got the heart-breaking call that they weren't going to offer him the job. In recalling that event, he was immediately sure this was what was connected to the need for anxiety in order to feel safe; his body felt better stuck in the house with anxiety than out in the world risking rejection. But I reminded him that emotions aren't logical, so we should be open to something that didn't make much sense. We checked by muscle testing the question *Was it the job heartbreak that caused me to feel like anxiety keeps me safe?* We got a "no." This is a great example of how, even though something makes great sense, it might not always be true.

Here are the questions we asked his body next. Remember, there is no specific formula for what to ask. We were just asking questions that we were wondering about consciously, and we knew his body would have the answers. Ask these questions with curiosity. Use whatever pops into your mind, as if you were trying to help a friend figure out where their issue came from.

Is this need for anxiety linked to work? We got a "no."

We pressed on. *Is this need for anxiety linked to family?* We got our "yes." *Is this need for anxiety linked to a specific person?* Again, a "yes."

We named off people in the family and finally got a "yes" connected to Ryan's Grandpa Ben. (Other things you could ask about are if an issue is connected to a place, health, career, or past relationships.)

Based on our new clue, I asked Ryan if he had any thoughts about how Grandpa Ben could be linked to anxiety making him feel safe. Basically, we were just trying to find what energies or issues were behind the belief that "anxiety keeps me safe." It's a simple game of guess and check. Ryan remembered only positive things about his grandpa. He shared that Grandpa Ben had been a high-powered attorney and had wanted Ryan to follow in his footsteps. While Ryan had planned to get his law degree, it was around age 22 that he decided to do something else. That's when his journey with anxiety began. But he remembered Grandpa Ben being very supportive of his decision and never giving him a hard time. Guess what, though? Through muscle testing, his body confirmed that Grandpa Ben's hope of him being an attorney was somehow linked to the root of anxiety— something he didn't even think was that big a deal! Remember, Ryan was convinced that his anxiety was linked to the company that had rejected him. The question we used to get to this conclusion was this: *Is this anxiety linked to Grandpa Ben hoping I'd be an attorney?* Simple!

Action Item: We used TTT to clear emotions around Grandpa Ben, *other people being unhappy with me,* and *chang-*

ing my mind without permission. These were all just random things that popped into our heads in relationship to Ryan's story. There was no specific formula for figuring them out. If anything comes up for you as you work with your story, clear them in this same way.

What we did next was talk about what we discovered. This is sort of a brainstorming process. Sometimes you'll come to a conclusion that makes sense and sometimes you have to just accept that it might not make sense.

What we ended up figuring out was that Ryan's main way to bond with his grandpa had been going to work with him. Growing up, Ryan had always thought his grandpa was so cool. They had talked about what it would be like when Ryan had an office like his, got to go to the courthouse, and so on. Somewhere in Ryan's subconscious, he had felt that if he didn't follow in Grandpa Ben's footsteps, he'd lose that relationship. More so, anxiety had made him feel safe because he'd felt that Grandpa Ben was more compassionate *because* he had anxiety. He might have even wondered how their relationship would be without it.

Action Item: Ryan had worried that he'd lose his relationship with Grandpa Ben if he didn't go into law. We used EFT and Chakra Tapping (about twenty minutes of each over two different sessions) to clear his feelings, fears, and insecurities around this belief. We tapped on the worry that was directly related to Grandpa Ben, but also tapped on another time when he'd been worried about losing a relationship with a friend who had pressured Ryan to join a basketball team that he had no interest in. In addition, Ryan also had the idea/belief that having anxiety was better or safer than disappointing people. We used The Sweep six times in a row to clear this.

Let me outline what we discovered about what was connected to Ryan's anxiety. This may seem like a lot of conflicting ideas and information to a beginner's eye, and it's true—it's a lot! But just take it step by step. Remember, there may be lots of different things from your past that are connected to the anxiety you're experiencing, but just go step by step, like Ryan and I did. We simply kept releasing the layers of energy as they came to us, whether the energies were tied up in a neat little package or not. It felt just as disorganized and all over the place to us as it might to you reading this, but we stayed focused on picking out the pieces that mattered.

Let's quickly review what Ryan and I worked with as a starting point. This was enough to help him see a big improvement in the anxiety in just a couple weeks.

- Ryan had the belief that "anxiety keeps me safe because it prevents me from having to be out in the world." We used The Sweep technique and repeated it four times until we used muscle testing to find out that the energy attached to this belief was completely gone.

- We used TTT to release about thirty stuck emotions from age 22.

- We also used TTT to clear emotions around Grandpa Ben, *other people being unhappy with me,* and *changing my mind without permission.*

- Ryan had worried that he'd lose his relationship with Grandpa Ben if he didn't go into law. We used EFT and Chakra Tapping to clear his feelings, fears, and insecurities around this belief.

- We tapped on the worry that was directly related to Grandpa Ben, but also tapped on another time when he'd been worried about losing a relationship with a friend who had pressured Ryan to join a basketball team that he had no interest in.

- Ryan believed that having anxiety was better or safer than disappointing people. We used The Sweep six times in a row to clear this. Typically The Sweep will clear a belief in a few rounds, but this one was extra stuck.

Again, there are dozens of different ways that we could have approached Ryan's situation, and all of them would have been perfectly fine! The great thing about this work, even if it makes you uncomfortable at first, is that there are no rules. Perhaps healing is even like an art form—however you go about creating your picture of health is just great.

Ryan saw a huge improvement in his anxiety in just the two weeks after our first few clearing sessions, and he continued to improve as he cleared more layers on his own.

As you know, there can be a lot of different energies contributing to anxiety that need to be cleared. That means healing is all about working from different angles at different times and in different ways. It's actually quite fun to solve the *puzzle* once you relax and get the hang of it.

Chapter Ten

* * * * * * * * * * * * * *

Advanced Clearing Practices

While you now have a solid understanding and foundation of how to clear anxiety, there are some advanced practices you might want to explore. All that you've learned thus far is complete and enough. However, these additional ways to use techniques may provide even more benefit to your healing. Specific areas of focus that we'll cover in this chapter include being energetically sensitive, anxiety triggered by reactions to food and more, and healing inherited and past-life energies.

I'm going to share with you how to address these issues using the techniques you already learned in previous chapters.

Energetic Sensitivity

Energetically sensitive people often absorb the energies of those around them, as we touched on in chapter 2. They may easily absorb and be affected by the emotions of others around them. This is not a defect in personality or anybody's fault. Some of us were just born into this world as sensitive souls, and it is in our nature to be empathic—maybe even to our detriment. Much of this pattern, though, happens on a subconscious level. We may naturally feel emotions more intensely and be affected by them more deeply than others in our family and our circle of friends. If you are easily overwhelmed or feel anxious around other people, you may be energetically sensitive.

Everything we've done up until this point has been important for strengthening your own energy field and feeling more at ease in life. The more of your own emotions and beliefs that you let go of, the less you will be affected by those around you. The reason for this is twofold. First, you will be clear enough that you don't "match up" with everyone else's emotional baggage. Second, your entire energy system will be stronger, which will help you be less affected by people around you. Here are a few targeted ideas to work with using the techniques that you already know. Feel free to expand on these ideas.

Release Stuck Emotions Using Thymus Test and Tap (TTT)

- Release stuck emotions *triggering energetic sensitivity.*
- Release stuck emotions *I've absorbed from others.*

Clear Unprocessed Experiences Using EFT or Chakra Tapping

- Clear experiences from your past where you felt responsible for the happiness of others.
- Clear experiences from your past where you know you took on the emotions or problems of others.

Change Harmful Beliefs Using The Sweep

- Clear *I'm too delicate* and install *I'm strong.*
- Clear *Everyone else has more power over me than I have over myself* and install *I'm empowered.*
- Clear *It is my job to carry the emotions of others* and install *I'm only responsible for my own emotions.*

Address Unhealthy Patterns

- Use The Sweep to clear *this old pattern of taking on everyone else's stuff* and install *I have healthy energetic boundaries.*

Helpful Tapping Scripts

- Being Triggered by Others (in the appendix)
- I'm Too Sensitive (in the appendix)

Negative Energetic Reactions to Foods, Substances, and Other Triggers

Many people are surprised to find out that anxiety can be triggered by negative reactions to things they come in contact with every single day. Just as you can have an allergic reaction to foods, scents, dust, or other substances, your body can actually have a negative energetic reaction too. A negative energetic reaction just means that your body's energy system has decided that a specific energy is dangerous for you (when really it's not). Because everything is really just energy, these reactions can happen in relationship to anything in your environment, including people, places, and things. Energetically speaking, the negative reaction comes from your body being overreactive or defensive about whatever you are coming into contact with. I have worked with people who have negative energetic reactions to their mother, a specific color or smell, the sun, and more!

This type of reaction can happen because at some point in your past you came into contact with a person, place, or thing *while* you were feeling a strong emotion or a high level of stress—either related or not related directly to it. Let me show you how this dynamic plays out.

Take the example of a stressful business meeting, as this is one I've seen countless times (although this could be a family gathering or any other type of event). Everyone is sitting around drinking coffee when suddenly someone starts ranting about their political views. As this is happening, you are drinking your latte with whipped cream, just trying to keep your rage to yourself, because this conversation reminds you of family disputes of the past over politics. As the situation unfolds and your own emotions come up, your body starts to become defensive and stressed.

While the memories of your past and the threat of a fight between you and your coworker are what's being activated or triggered, your body decides to blame the coffee you are drinking, because that's what you are in direct contact with at the time. Your energy system then creates a program to "react" to coffee so that you will be protected from this stress in the future. Or maybe it doesn't link the coffee but instead "blames" the perfume you can smell of the coworker sitting next to you, so you then become reactive to perfume. If your system perceives that something like this is a danger to you, it can create a negative reaction in an effort to keep you away from it in the future. It's simply a misdirected protection mechanism. Note: Allergic reactions are considered a medical condition and can be very serious. Do not use this approach in any way that puts you at risk.

How to Clear an Energetic Reaction in the Body
A lot of negative energetic reactions will clear on their own as you work on stuck emotions, unprocessed experiences, and harmful beliefs. However, you can target them directly as well.

Step 1: Identify the Reaction
First, you'll want to identify what's causing the reaction in your body, if you don't already know. While there is no sure way to

figure this out, a lot of guessing and muscle testing will usually work.

Using muscle testing, ask, *Is _____ (person, place, or thing) causing a negative reaction in my body?*

Once you narrow down the cause of the reaction to a person, place, or thing, here are some more specific ideas you can try:

- Fluorescent lights
- Your mother, brother, sister, etc.
- Certain smells
- Specific foods
- Trees, grasses, flowers, etc.

Step 2: Clear the Reaction

Once you know what your body is reacting to, you'll want to clear any stuck emotions, unprocessed experiences, or harmful beliefs that are associated with the cause. Here are some ideas of how to do that. Feel free to muscle-test to see which techniques (or maybe all of them) might be beneficial for you.

Release Stuck Emotions Using Thymus Test and Tap (TTT):

- Release stuck emotions *triggering negative reactions to _____.*
- Release stuck emotions *causing my body to be overreactive and defensive.* This is a general approach and is especially helpful if you have a lot of negative reactions to clear.

Clear Unprocessed Experiences Using EFT or Chakra Tapping:

- Clear any unprocessed experiences that may be linked to the reaction. In the previous example I shared, the experience might be a past fight that you had with family members about their political views.

Change Harmful Beliefs Using The Sweep:

- Change harmful beliefs such as *Coffee is dangerous for me.* Then install something like *Coffee is safe for me.*

- Clear the harmful belief *My body has to protect me from _____.* Then install *My body can process _____ with ease.*

Other:

- Use The Sweep to clear *this negative reaction to _____.* Then install *I can be safe around _____.*

Helpful Tapping Script:

- Use the Clear Energetic Negative Reactions tapping script (in the appendix).

Step 3: Check Your Work

After you've done the clearing, it's a good idea to check back and muscle-test to see if the reaction is gone. While I've worked with many clients to clear major reactions successfully, again, do not use this process to address anything you are highly reactive to.

Tip: I don't want you to be scared that every time you feel stressed, you'll create negative reactions to everything around you. That's the whole point of all the work we're doing—to release the old and also begin new patterns of feeling our emotions while allowing them to move out of the body. Everything we've been doing up until now has been helping to bring the body into a calm and relaxed state so that our system can better handle both internal stress and the world around us. It can be very helpful to use the following trick the first few times you come into contact with something after using the clearing protocol to clear it. For example, if you are going to eat dairy after clearing energetic reactions to it, simply tap through your EFT points for one minute before you eat it and one minute after. You don't need to say anything as you tap. This will help your body be in the most balanced place when you ingest it and also as you metabolize it. You only need to do this the first two or three times after clearing.

Inherited Energies

Inherited energies (sometimes called generational energies) can be any type of emotional baggage that you've already been working with: stuck emotions, unprocessed experiences, or harmful beliefs. The only difference in the case of these inherited energies is that they've been passed down to you instead of accumulated during your own lifetime. Just like DNA is passed down the family line, emotional energies are too. We are seeing increasing evidence of the definitive effect of one generation's trauma on those that come after it.

If you're being affected by inherited energy, you may feel as if "heavy" or "dark" energy has been following you your whole life, or you may see that your parents and grandparents are struggling with challenges that are similar to yours. Most people have inherited energy, but I see this even more often in families with heavy energy lineages like Holocaust survivors, such as in my own family. If you resonate with the idea of inherited energy, it's worth exploring.

While most of my own ancestors were killed in the Holocaust, my paternal grandparents, along with my uncle (who was a little boy at the time), survived. In each of them, the trauma was apparent in different ways. Even though my dad wasn't born until a couple years after the war ended, he struggled with depression throughout his life. When I recognized the magnitude of what had happened to my family, I began to study the effects of generational trauma. I do think addressing inherited energy was an important part of my own overall healing.

It's important to know that generational energies are very, very common. I don't think any of us got to this lifetime without them. Our lineage is part of who we are, and just like we received many good traits and probably positive energy from our ancestors, we probably also ended up with some stuff we don't want. There is no reason to be angry with your family about this. Just focus on releasing it so you can move forward. The really cool part about doing generational work is that I believe that these energies keep getting passed down until they reach a person who is evolved and conscious enough to be capable of clearing them. You are that person! What a great chance this is for you to break familial patterns.

How to Clear Inherited Energies

Working with inherited energy is done using the same techniques you use for yourself. Hooray, because you already know them all! The only difference is that we are focusing on energy that did not originate in our lifetime.

You don't do anything different to clear inherited/generational energy than what you'd do if it was your own, because in essence it is your energy now. The only thing you need to do is "call it out" as inherited energy so your subconscious knows exactly what to help you clear. That phrasing is incorporated in my directions about how to clear.

Here are some general ideas on clearing inherited energies, but you may find your own ways to do this too. As always, feel free to muscle-test to determine which techniques will be most beneficial for you.

Release Stuck Emotions Using Thymus Test and Tap (TTT):

- Release inherited stuck emotions in the same way you would release regular stuck emotions, but call out *inherited stuck emotions* either vocally when you muscle-test to find emotions to release from the list or by holding the intention to find inherited emotions.

Clear Unprocessed Experiences Using EFT or Chakra Tapping:

One way to find out about unprocessed experiences is by using what you know about your family history. What stories have you heard that you imagine were traumatic? What might have been passed down to you?

- Identify inherited energies: It's always helpful to muscle-test to help identify inherited energies that would be beneficial to release. To do this, you could ask a series of questions:

  ◆ *Do I have inherited/generational stuck emotions contributing to anxiety?* If you do, follow the directions below.

  ◆ *Do I have an inherited unprocessed experience contributing to anxiety?* Here you are asking if an experience (and its energy) was passed down to you from one of your ancestors. If you get a "yes," it can be helpful to know which side of your ancestry it came from—your mother's or your father's. Once you identify that through muscle testing, think back to or do some family research about some family experiences that might still be stuck in your ancestral line (for example, experiencing depression associated with a car accident, losing a child in the family, etc.). If you can't identify the specific experience(s), don't worry. You can use the general approach outlined below with The Sweep technique, or use the tapping script I created for this (which you can find in the appendix).

- Sweep out general inherited energy: Even if you don't know what inherited energy is affecting you, you can still clear it. This is something you'd repeat over and over again during your healing journey, and not just do once and forget about it. Use The Sweep to clear *this inherited energy that no longer serves me* and install *I can move on now*.

- Clear any inherited unprocessed experiences you may be carrying from your ancestors in the exact same way you would for yourself, but incorporate the phrase *this experience from my ancestors*. For example, for the first part of your set-up statement, you could use *Even though I have been carrying this experience from my ancestors, …* You can use some of the wording you'd use with subconscious tapping since you likely won't have concrete details to work with (but your subconscious mind will).

Change Harmful Beliefs Using The Sweep:
If you can identify a message or belief that your family seems to have, you can clear it using The Sweep. If you want to use muscle testing, ask, *Do I have an inherited harmful belief contributing to anxiety?* If so, try to identify the belief (or beliefs). This can actually be a really fun process! Think of the things you've heard members of your family say that might be their belief but not actually the truth. Some examples are "Money

doesn't grow on trees," "No pain, no gain," and "Life's not fair." I'll explain the clearing process next. Muscle testing is optional in this one because most people can use their conscious mind to come up with plenty of beliefs to work with.

- Change inherited harmful beliefs by revising the first part of The Sweep script to *Even though I have this inherited belief that* _____, …

Other:

- Use The Sweep to clear *this inherited energy that no longer serves me* and install *I can move on from my family's past now.*

A Helpful Tapping Script:

- Use the Release Inherited Energies tapping script (in the appendix).

Other Triggers for Anxiety

Almost anything can be a trigger for anxiety—which means, thankfully, clearing those things can make a positive difference. Oftentimes we can find some important triggers and clear them if we look at what was happening when we started to feel bad. Most people with anxiety will look at obvious things, like if someone upset them or they felt scared or upset in some obvious way, but the truth is that many things have a propensity to trigger us. Here are a few I see all the time that might be useful to work on releasing. I'll explain them and then give you specific ways to address them directly following.

Times of Day

Sometimes a specific time of day (morning, afternoon, night, or even something as targeted as 3:00 p.m.) can be a trigger. Several years ago, I realized I was having a very hard time in the morning. Now, I've never been a cheery morning person, but this was different. I kept waking up feeling heavy and teary-eyed. Then, by around 11:00 a.m., I'd spontaneously be totally fine and back to my normal happy self. This made me look at the mornings in a whole new way. What I realized was that because my dad had passed away in the morning, perhaps I still had some energy around that was being activated at that time of day. I used muscle testing to ask my body, and lo and behold, it was indeed affecting me. Here are a few things I cleared: the harmful belief that *the morning is dangerous*, the unprocessed experience of waiting around in the morning until my dad finally passed, and stuck emotions *triggered by the morning.*

Seasons and Weather

Our memories get connected to all kinds of things, and seasons and weather are some of the big ones! Just think about big events from your past. Do you remember the dark sky or the clouds or snow when a certain event happened? Maybe you remember feeling good sitting in the summer sun at the beach when you got that call from your boss that you lost your job, or maybe you just feel blue during certain seasons or when certain weather patterns happen. Whatever negative connotations you have with seasons and/or weather, you can clear them.

How to Clear Energies Connected to Specific Times of Day, Seasons, and Weather Patterns

Here are some general protocols for clearing energies around specific times of day, seasons, and weather patterns.

Release Stuck Emotions Using Thymus Test and Tap (TTT)

- Release stuck emotions *triggered or activated by* _____ *(a specific time of day, season, or weather pattern).*

Clear Unprocessed Experiences Using EFT or Chakra Tapping

- Clear experiences from your past when something upsetting happened at a specific time of day, during a specific season, or amidst the same kind of weather that's affecting you now. For example, if you remember hearing your parents fight every night after you went to bed, then *nighttime* might be a time of day that still holds energy for you. If you lost your job on a bright summer day, you might have issues with the summer.

Change Harmful Beliefs Using The Sweep

- Clear *This* _____ *(time of day, season, or type of weather) is dangerous for me.*

Other

- Use The Sweep to clear *any negative energy around* _____ *(time of day, season, or weather)* and install _____ *(time of day, season, or weather) can be positive for me.*

Helpful Tapping Scripts

- Use the Clear Negative Energetic Reactions tapping script in the appendix and revise the wording to fit your specific clearing needs.

You now have a great new set of protocols for clearing in an advanced way. If you play around with these ideas, I'm sure you'll come up with a lot more that could be beneficial for you to work with. The sky is truly the limit!

By learning and using my energetic approach to working with anxiety, you are a more empowered person than when you first began. While anxiety may have always seemed like something totally out of your control, you now understand that doesn't have to be your reality. There is no one right way to heal anxiety, but I will promise you that making sure *you* are an integral part of your healing is absolutely necessary.

Do not become overwhelmed by the vastness of what you have learned in this book. Remember that using these tools in tiny baby steps for a few minutes a day, or only utilizing a couple of the techniques you resonate with most, can be enough to change your life. *You* are enough to change your life. And while I can't say that it will always be easy, it *is* possible. And worth it. *You* are worth it. Happy healing, my new friend. You've got this.

Tapping Scripts

Part of the success that comes from tapping is due to your script addressing your own feelings and thoughts. However, I hope the following tapping scripts give you a great starting point and help you gain new ideas for your own clearing. For these scripts to be most effective, change and revise whatever phrases you need to so they apply to your specific situation.

You will need to repeat these scripts several times in a row, check in and see how you're feeling, and repeat as many times as necessary. As I mentioned when you first learned EFT in chapter 5, it's unlikely that doing only one or two rounds of tapping will provide much benefit. So feel free to go through the scripts again and again, and if prompted with your own ideas, make sure to incorporate those phrases.

If one or more of these scripts really resonates with you, feel free to use it even multiple times a day. As you already know about tapping, consistency (and persistence) is key! If having these scripts to follow helps you do the work consistently, then go for it.

List of Tapping Scripts

Clear Negative Energetic Reactions
Release Inherited Energies
Ease Processing Discomfort
Anxious but Don't Know Why
Feeling Out of Control
Calm the Fight, Flight, or Freeze Response
Being Triggered by Others
I'm Too Sensitive

Which Tapping Points to Use

As you know by now, EFT and Chakra Tapping are both great techniques for healing anxiety! Which one you use depends completely on which one you feel you get better results from, or what you feel most drawn to use as you're getting ready to tap. I often use both. I switch off—a few rounds of EFT points, then a few rounds of Chakra Tapping points.

> ***A Note about the Extra EFT Tapping Point (Gamut Point):*** Remember the gamut point (top of the hand) you learned that you can add in and use with EFT? If you're pretty comfortable with EFT now, try incorporating this point more and see how it feels. Again, I do use it, but I add it to my tapping rounds on a more intuitive basis than as a consistent practice.
>
> As a reminder, when you get to the gamut point, you're going to do the following routine to help you further release trauma and integrate healing by engaging the right and left hemispheres of the brain using eye movements. Continue tapping the top of the hand point while you do the following:

Close your eyes, open your eyes, shift your eyes down and to the right (don't move your head), shift your eyes down and to the left (don't move your head), roll your eyes in a big circle in front of you, then roll them in the other direction, hum a few seconds of a song (anything will do!), count to five quickly out loud (1, 2, 3, 4, 5), and then hum for a few more seconds.

How to Use the Tapping Scripts

Whether you choose EFT or Chakra Tapping, you'll be using the same format for each script:

- First, you always begin by saying the set-up statement while tapping continuously on the karate chop point. You can either choose one of the set-up statements I suggest and repeat it three times or use all three of the set-up statements I provide and say each of them once.

- Next, you'll tap through the rest of the points for several rounds (as many as you need to feel better). When doing this, you can use either the EFT points or the Chakra Tapping points to continue with the script and tap through the points in order, from the top of the head back to the karate chop point. I have not noted in the script what specific phrases to say at what points. Instead, I have listed suggested phrases for all the rest of the points so you can simply go through them in order.

- Finally, you'll come to the final round of positive tapping. This round should not be done until you're ready to wind down your session. You should do the final round of positive tapping so you rotate through all the tapping points once, just to end your session.

Script: **Clear Negative Energetic Reactions**

Remember that anxiety can be triggered by negative reactions to common things you come in contact with every single day. If you can be aware of when you feel triggered into anxiety, you can decipher what energies around you might be playing a part in that. This tapping script can help you start addressing and calming those reactions in your body. You will want to use the tapping scripts consistently to break long-held or intense reactions.

Step 1: Use the Set-Up Statement While Tapping the Karate Chop Point

Begin by saying the set-up statement while tapping continuously on the karate chop point. You can either choose one of the following set-up statements and repeat it three times or use all three of the statements and say each of them once.

> *Even though I have this reaction to _____,*
> *I choose to change that pattern.*
>
> *Even though my body can't yet handle _____,*
> *I can be okay anyway.*
>
> *Even though my body doesn't like _____,*
> *it's safe to release that energy.*

Step 2: Tap Through the Rest of the Points

Next, use either the EFT points or the Chakra Tapping points to continue with the script and tap through the points in order, from the top of the head back to the karate chop point. Do as many rounds as you need until you feel better.

I have given you several phrases to use. I suggest using one phrase for each tapping point, rotating through the list of phrases over and over again until you're ready to stop tapping.

Remember to work in your own words and phrases as they come to you.

My body doesn't like _____.

My body is really scared of _____.

For some reason my body doesn't like _____.

This strong reaction to _____.

My body got the idea that this _____ is scary!

This _____ is dangerous for me.

My body can't handle _____.

This strong reaction to _____.

My body doesn't like _____.

My body is really scared of _____.

For some reason my body doesn't like _____.

I'm so reactive to _____.

My body can't seem to handle _____.

Step 3: Do a Final Round of Positive Tapping
When you're feeling better, do a final round of positive tapping for a minimum of one round (or once, through all of the points).

I'm ready to be friends with _____ now.

I can be perfectly okay with _____.

My body can relax around _____ now.

I'm willing to create a new pattern now.

All can be well now.

I can easily handle _____ now.

I'm okay.

I can feel at ease with _____.
It's time to relax.
I can be okay.
_____ and I can coexist now.
I'm safe around _____ now.
I'm okay.

When you're done clearing your negative energetic reactions, it's important to know whether they really have been completely cleared. The best way to confirm that your work is done is to muscle-test again. I typically use this testing statement: *This _____ is 100 percent safe for me now.* Once you get a "yes" response from the body, the person, place, or thing should no longer cause a negative reaction for you. If possible, it's beneficial to wait twenty-four hours before coming into contact with the source of the reactive energy again.

In addition and as a reminder, the next time you do come in contact with the source of the reactive energy, I suggest that you use your EFT tapping points to tap for about one minute before and after contact. You don't need to say anything, but rather just tap the points while in the presence of that energy in order to help reinforce the calm and balanced state. This typically needs to be done only with the first few contacts after clearing.

> **Note:** Again, as a reminder, this practice is for use with negative energetic reactions. Allergies are a medical condition. Please use common sense and caution when addressing any type of reaction and don't rely on this practice for your health or safety.

Script: **Release Inherited Energies**

Inherited (or generational) energies can be any type of emotional baggage that's been passed down to you from your ancestors. Even though this type of energy is not technically "yours" in terms of originating in your body, it can still have a big impact on you. This script is a great way to release inherited energy, even if you don't know where or whom it came from or specifically what it is.

Step 1: Use the Set-Up Statement While Tapping the Karate Chop Point

Begin by saying the set-up statement while tapping continuously on the karate chop point. You can either choose one of the following set-up statements and repeat it three times or use all three of the statements and say each of them once.

> *Even though I have this inherited energy stuck in my body,*
> *I can be okay anyway.*
> *Even though I'm carrying the energy of my ancestors,*
> *it's time to let it go.*
> *Even though I may have inherited energy that's causing anxiety, I'm ready to move on.*

Step 2: Tap Through the Rest of the Points

Next, use either the EFT points or the Chakra Tapping points to continue with the script and tap through the points in order, from the top of the head back to the karate chop point. Do as many rounds as you need until you feel better.

I have given you several phrases to use. I suggest using one phrase for each tapping point, rotating through the list of phrases over and over again until you're ready to stop tapping.

Remember to work in your own words and phrases as they come to you.

I'm holding this old energy that's not mine.

My body is being affected by this inherited anxiety.

For some reason my body is carrying my ancestors' energies.

This inherited anxiety might be contributing to anxiety.

It might be making it hard for me to feel safe.

This energy isn't even mine.

This inherited energy is stuck in my body.

This energy that no longer serves me.

My body doesn't need to hold this old generational anxiety any longer.

My body has carried it for so long.

These inherited energies in my body.

They're not even mine to carry.

Step 3: Do a Final Round of Positive Tapping

Once you're feeling better, do a final round of positive tapping for a minimum of one round (or once, through all of the points).

I honor my body for holding this inherited energy.

I'm ready to let it go now.

I'm healing for all of my family now.

I can heal these old energies now.

I can move forward.

It's time to let go.

I'm ready to let it go now.

It's time for me to heal.

I am free from this old energy.

My family is free now too.

I healed it for all of us.

I'm healing.

I'm okay now.

Script: **Ease Processing Discomfort**

During and after energy work, remember that you are shifting and rebalancing your energy. You might recall from earlier that we call this time period "processing." Your body and its energy field (which extends far beyond your actual physical body) are simply going through an adjustment process. Not everyone feels these shifts as discomfort or even at all. However, if you do feel them, I've provided you with this tapping script. In addition, it helps to do some grounding and drink extra water, as being ungrounded and/or dehydrated will make it difficult for your body's energies to adjust. You should take a break from doing big clearings for a day or so until your body catches up.

Step 1: Use the Set-Up Statement While Tapping the Karate Chop Point

Begin by saying the set-up statement while tapping continuously on the karate chop point. You can either choose one of the following set-up statements and repeat it three times or use all three of the statements and say each of them once.

Even though I feel worse right now,
I choose to let this energy move through me.

Even though I feel _____ (explain how you feel),
I can be okay anyway.

Even though I'm not feeling well, I can be okay.

Step 2: Tap Through the Rest of the Points

Next, use either the EFT points or the Chakra Tapping points to continue with the script and tap through the points in order, from the top of the head back to the karate chop point. Do as many rounds as you need until you feel better.

I have given you several phrases to use. I suggest using one phrase for each tapping point, rotating through the list of phrases over and over again until you're ready to stop tapping. Remember to work in your own words and phrases as they come to you.

> **Note:** To ease processing discomfort, it's essential that you explain exactly how you feel here. Be sure to be specific, and feel free to "vent" through all of the points using your own descriptions of how you feel, even if they deviate from this script.

I'm feeling so _____ (describe your symptoms, emotional or physical).

I just feel off.

I feel this discomfort in my _____.

Feeling very _____ (hopeless, tired, weird, etc.).

I'm feeling all of these old emotions moving.

So much has been stuck for so long.

My body is really feeling the shift.

It doesn't feel good at all.

It's making me _____ (anxious, frustrated, etc.).

This processing is making me feel _____.

I hope this goes away soon.

I'm not sure what to do.

I feel _____.

Step 3: Do a Final Round of Positive Tapping

When you're feeling better, do a final round of positive tapping for a minimum of one round (or once, through all of the points).

I can let this energy move through me.

I can process with ease.

Processing will get easier and easier for me.

My body is already moving this energy out.

It's only going to get better from here.

All of that old energy is leaving my energy field.

I'm just feeling off because of that.

I can process with ease.

I'm okay now.

My body can relax now.

Script: **Anxious but Don't Know Why**

When we're feeling really anxious, it can be hard to focus on doing anything to help ourselves feel better. This tapping script is perfect when you are feeling too unsettled to do the deeper work of addressing stuck emotions, unprocessed experiences, and harmful beliefs. This script will help you shift enough energy to then be able to use the foundational approach you learned in this book.

Step 1: Use the Set-Up Statement While Tapping the Karate Chop Point

Begin by saying the set-up statement while tapping continuously on the karate chop point. You can either choose one of the following set-up statements and repeat it three times or use all three of the statements and say each of them once.

Even though I'm feeling _____ (explain how you feel) mostly in my _____ (describe how it feels in your body, if you feel it there), I can relax now.

Even though I feel so unsettled and terrible, I can let it go now.

Even though I might be feeling anxious about _____ (see if you can identify something triggering you in general), I choose to release it.

Step 2: Tap Through the Rest of the Points

Next, use either the EFT points or the Chakra Tapping points to continue with the script and tap through the points in order, from the top of the head back to the karate chop point. Do as many rounds as you need until you feel better.

I have given you several phrases to use. I suggest using one phrase for each tapping point, rotating through the list of phrases over and over again until you're ready to stop tapping. Remember to work in your own words and phrases as they come to you.

I just can't relax.

Something feels off.

I feel it in my _____ (name the part of the body).

I'm not even sure what is upsetting me.

I don't know what to do.

I just keep thinking about _____.

It makes me so anxious.

I'm so tired of feeling this way.

I feel so _____.

Things feel out of my control.

I hate that I don't know why I feel this way.

I feel so _____.

This anxiety is taking over.

Step 3: Do a Final Round of Positive Tapping

When you're feeling better, do a final round of positive tapping for a minimum of one round (or once, through all of the points).

I can let this energy move through me.

My body is already moving this energy out.

All of that old energy is leaving my energy field.

I'm ready to let go now.

I can relax now.

I can be calm now.

I'm releasing that old energy.

Everything can be okay.

Relaxing…

It's safe to relax now.

I'm okay now.

All is well.

I'm safe.

Script: Feeling Out of Control

So many of us grew up believing that if we could only be in control, everything would be okay. This tapping script is great for when you are having a hard time letting go of the need to control and are feeling anxious as a result.

Step 1: Use the Set-Up Statement While Tapping the Karate Chop Point

Begin by saying the set-up statement while tapping continuously on the karate chop point. You can either choose one of the following set-up statements and repeat it three times or use all three of the statements and say each of them once.

> *Even though I'm feeling out of control_____ (add any detail you can) mostly in my _____ (describe how it feels in your body, if you feel it there), I can be okay anyway.*
>
> *Even though I feel so unsettled and out of control, I can be okay anyway.*
>
> *Even though I feel anxious when I can't control things like _____ (give examples of what kinds of things come to mind), I can be okay anyway.*

Step 2: Tap Through the Rest of the Points

Next, use either the EFT points or the Chakra Tapping points to continue with the script and tap through the points in order, from the top of the head back to the karate chop point. Do as many rounds as you need until you feel better.

I have given you several phrases to use. I suggest using one phrase for each tapping point, rotating through the list of phrases over and over again until you're ready to stop tapping. Remember to work in your own words and phrases as they come to you.

> *I need to be in control.*
>
> *I feel so out of control.*
>
> *I feel it in my _____ (name the part of the body).*
>
> *I'd feel better if I was in control.*

I don't know what to do.

I just keep feeling like if I can't control things, then _____ will happen.

It makes me so anxious to be out of control.

I feel unsafe. (You can substitute this for something more targeted to you in the moment if you wish.)

I feel helpless. (You can substitute this for something more targeted to you in the moment if you wish.)

It feels terrible not to be able to change things.

I just want to feel in control.

I'm afraid that if I can't control this, then _____ will happen.

I feel so scared.

Step 3: Do a Final Round of Positive Tapping

When you're feeling better, do a final round of positive tapping for a minimum of one round (or once, through all of the points).

I'm ready to be okay now.

I can relax even when I'm not in control.

I can be calm now.

I'm going to be fine.

I can let go.

Letting go…

I'm safe.

All is well.

I'm safe.

I'm okay no matter what.

I can relax now.

I'm okay no matter what.

It's time to relax.

Script: **Calm the Fight, Flight, or Freeze Response**

As you learned in chapters 1 and 2, the fight, flight, or freeze response is a huge contributor of anxiety, causing your body to be in freak-out mode. This tapping script addresses the fight, flight, or freeze response in the body in order to help you calm down and heal.

Step 1: Use the Set-Up Statement While Tapping the Karate Chop Point

Begin by saying the set-up statement while tapping continuously on the karate chop point. You can either choose one of the following set-up statements and repeat it three times or use all three of the statements and say each of them once.

Even though I'm feeling very triggered now _____ (explain how you feel in detail if you can) and it feels _____ (describe how it feels in your body, if you feel it there), I choose to be calm.

Even though I feel so _____ (panicky, sweaty, etc.), I can be okay anyway.

Even though I know my fight, flight, or freeze response has been triggered, I give my body permission to calm down now.

Step 2: Tap Through the Rest of the Points

Next, use either the EFT points or the Chakra Tapping points to continue with the script and tap through the points in order, from the top of the head back to the karate chop point. Do as many rounds as you need until you feel better.

I have given you several phrases to use. I suggest using one phrase for each tapping point, rotating through the list of phrases over and over again until you're ready to stop tapping. Remember to work in your own words and phrases as they come to you.

I just feel so triggered. (If you can identify another emotion such as fearful, nervous, etc., that's great.)

I feel _____ (shaken, nervous, etc.).

I feel it in my _____ (name the part of the body).

I'm not sure what happened. (If you are sure, then use *I think _____ is what triggered me.*)

My body is just so riled up now.

I just keep thinking _____.

It makes me so anxious.

This reminds me of when _____.

I felt so _____.

I feel _____.

All of this anxiety in my body.

My body is in freak-out mode.

It's hard to calm down.

Step 3: Do a Final Round of Positive Tapping

When you're feeling better, do a final round of positive tapping for a minimum of one round (or once, through all of the points).

I'm ready to calm down now.

I can relax now.

My body can calm down now.

I'm releasing that old energy.

Everything can be okay.

Relaxing…

It's safe to relax now.

I'm okay now.

All is well.

I'm safe.

It's okay to allow my body to relax.

I'm safe.

I'm secure.

Script: Being Triggered by Others

It is common (and easy) to allow others to trigger us, especially since we have no control of other people. This script is a great way to release energy when someone you love—or someone you don't even know—triggers you.

Step 1: Use the Set-Up Statement While Tapping the Karate Chop Point

Begin by saying the set-up statement while tapping continuously on the karate chop point. You can either choose one of the following set-up statements and repeat it three times or use all three of the statements and say each of them once.

> *Even though I'm feeling very triggered by _____
> (insert the person's name or describe the group of people
> if that applies; for example, "my family" or "all the happy
> people on Facebook") and it feels _____ (describe how
> you feel, perhaps left out, angry, etc.), I choose to reclaim
> my own energy.*

Even though I feel so _____ (sad, frustrated, etc.) because _____ (describe why you think you're being triggered), I can be okay anyway.

Even though I'm so triggered, I give my body permission to calm down now.

Step 2: Tap Through the Rest of the Points

Next, use either the EFT points or the Chakra Tapping points to continue with the script and tap through the points in order, from the top of the head back to the karate chop point. Do as many rounds as you need until you feel better.

I have given you several phrases to use. I suggest using one phrase for each tapping point, rotating through the list of phrases over and over again until you're ready to stop tapping. Remember to work in your own words and phrases as they come to you.

I just feel so triggered because _____. (Why do you think this is affecting you like it is?)

I feel it in my _____ (describe where you feel it in your body, if that applies).

I'm so _____ (describe how you feel).

When other people _____ (disregard my feelings, ignore me, don't let me talk, etc.), I get so upset.

My body is just so triggered right now.

I'm worried that _____ (I'll never calm down, so-and-so will be mad at me forever, etc.).

It makes me so anxious.

This reminds me of when _____.

I felt so _____.

I feel _____.

All of this anxiety because _____ (person's name or reference to group of people) triggered me.

My body is really freaking out about this.

It's hard to let it go.

Step 3: Do a Final Round of Positive Tapping

When you're feeling better, do a final round of positive tapping for a minimum of one round (or once, through all of the points).

I'm ready to let it go now.

I can relax even if _____ (state the worst-case scenario, like "Bob will never forgive me").

My body can relax now.

I'm releasing all of this adrenaline.

I trust that I can be okay no matter what.

Relaxing…

It's okay.

I'm fine no matter what.

Relaxing…

It's okay if my relationships aren't perfect.

I can be okay anyway.

All is well.

I'm secure.

Script: **I'm Too Sensitive**

If you are energetically sensitive, you might find that you feel triggered right, left, and center. This can be really frustrating and disheartening, but I promise that by doing all the work in this book, your system will become stronger than ever. If you seem to feel emotions more intensely than those around you do, you may be energetically sensitive. This script, especially if used often, will help you to be less affected by the world around you and more centered in your own wonderful energy field.

Step 1: Use the Set-Up Statement While Tapping the Karate Chop Point

Begin by saying the set-up statement while tapping continuously on the karate chop point. You can either choose one of the following set-up statements and repeat it three times or use all three of the statements and say each of them once.

Even though I sometimes feel like a sponge for the world around me, I choose to reclaim my own energy.

Even though I feel so thrown off by things and like I can't handle life, I choose to change this pattern.

Even though I'm so sensitive, I give my body permission to feel strong and centered.

Step 2: Tap Through the Rest of the Points

Next, use either the EFT points or the Chakra Tapping points to continue with the script and tap through the points in order, from the top of the head back to the karate chop point. Do as many rounds as you need until you feel better.

I have given you several phrases to use. I suggest using one phrase for each tapping point, rotating through the list of phrases over and over again until you're ready to stop tapping. Remember to work in your own words and phrases as they come to you.

I feel so sensitive.

I feel like other people can handle things so easily.

Why me?

Sometimes I feel like a sponge for the world.

Maybe my body has a habit of taking everything on.

I want to feel more centered and protected.

It makes me so anxious to be sensitive like this.

My body's pattern of taking everything on.

This energetic sensitivity.

I feel so sensitive.

I wish I could feel strong and stable no matter what is happening.

My body really gets shaken up by the world around me.

It's hard for me to stay in my own energy field.

Step 3: Do a Final Round of Positive Tapping

When you're feeling better, do a final round of positive tapping for a minimum of one round (or once, through all of the points).

I can feel strong and grounded.

Even if I feel everything, I don't have to take it on.

I can have a protected energy field.

I'm strong and protected.

I can learn to take on only what's mine.

I'm resilient.

I'm safe.

I'm okay no matter what.

Feeling protected…

I'm safe.

I can be okay .

All is well.

I'm secure.

* * * * * * * * * * * * * * *

Discussion Questions for Support Groups, Book Clubs, and Organizations

1. Is there any way in which anxiety serves you? What might you miss about anxiety when you overcome it? (These questions require some big-time bravery to answer them honestly.)

2. If you could frame your journey with anxiety as a book, what would the title be?

3. What was your aha moment in the book? Why?

4. Is there anything you disagree with or don't resonate with from the book? Why?

5. What line or part of the book do you want as a sticky note by your desk or bed?

6. Did this book change your perspective on healing or just confirm what you already believe or know?

7. What parts of the book have you found yourself thinking about the most?

8. What technique is your favorite or helps you feel the most empowered? Why?

9. Whom do you wish would read this book that you know won't? Why won't they and why do you think they should?

10. Which parts or techniques are you most likely to teach to a loved one? Whom do you most want to share this with most, and why?

11. If you could ask Amy one question, what would it be?

12. If you'd read this book earlier, do you think it would have changed your path in life?

Amy loves talking with readers about her books and work. If you are part of a book club or other group that is reading this together, feel free to contact Amy through her website (www. amybscher.com) to arrange an in-person or Skype visit.

* * * * * * * * * * * * * * *

Index

To Write to the Author

If you wish to contact the author or would like more information about this book, please write to the author in care of Llewellyn Worldwide Ltd. and we will forward your request. Both the author and the publisher appreciate hearing from you and learning of your enjoyment of this book and how it has helped you. Llewellyn Worldwide Ltd. cannot guarantee that every letter written to the author can be answered, but all will be forwarded. Please write to:

Amy B. Scher
⁄ Llewellyn Worldwide
2143 Wooddale Drive
Woodbury, MN 55125-2989

Please enclose a self-addressed stamped envelope for reply,
or $1.00 to cover costs. If outside the U.S.A., enclose
an international postal reply coupon.

Many of Llewellyn's authors have websites with additional information and resources. For more information, please visit our website at http://www.llewellyn.com.

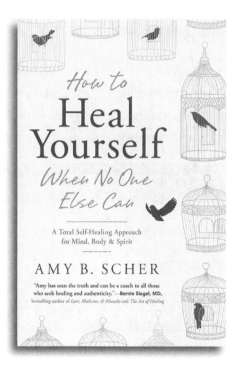

How to
Heal
Yourself
When No One
Else Can

A Total Self-Healing Approach
for Mind, Body & Spirit

AMY B. SCHER

"Amy has seen the truth and can be a coach to all those
who seek healing and authenticity." —**Bernie Siegel, MD,**
bestselling author of *Love, Medicine, & Miracles* and *The Art of Healing*

How to Heal Yourself When No One Else Can
A Total Self-Healing Approach for Mind, Body & Spirit
Amy B. Scher

Using energy therapy and emotional healing techniques, *How to Heal Yourself When No One Else Can* shows you how to love, accept, and be yourself no matter what. Energy therapist Amy B. Scher presents a down-to-earth three-part approach to removing blockages, changing your relationship with stress, and coming into alignment with who you truly are.

After overcoming late-stage chronic Lyme disease, Amy came to an important epiphany that healing is much more than just physical. Her dramatic story of healing serves as a powerful example of how beneficial it is to address our emotional energies, particularly when nothing else works. Discover the four main areas of imbalance and the easy ways to address them on your journey to complete and permanent healing. With Amy's guidance, you can get rid of blocks you never knew you had and finally move forward. Whether you are experiencing physical symptoms or are just feeling lost, sad, anxious, or emotionally unbalanced—this book can improve your wellbeing and your life.

978-0-7387-4554-1, 288 pp., 6 x 9   **$17.99**

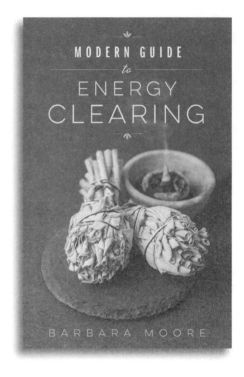

MODERN GUIDE
to
ENERGY
CLEARING

BARBARA MOORE

Modern Guide to Energy Clearing

Barbara Moore

This book is a complete guide to transforming your life by working with energy. Discover how to clear inappropriate energy and how to maintain healthy energy in yourself, your home, your workplace, and other shared or public spaces. Explore techniques for personal clearing, cording, shielding, supporting the spirit of a place, clearing clutter, setting intentions, and addressing the elements.

Like any kind of hygiene, spiritual wellbeing depends on consistent attention and good habits. *Modern Guide to Energy Clearing* provides the basic techniques you need to create a life of peace and abundance.

978-0-7387-5349-2, 240 pp., 5 ¹/₄ x 8   **$16.99**

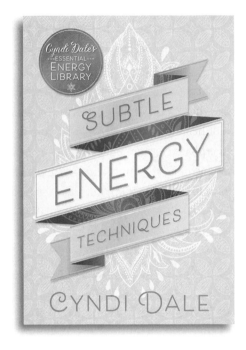

Cyndi Dale's
···ESSENTIAL···
ENERGY
LIBRARY

SUBTLE

ENERGY

TECHNIQUES

CYNDI DALE

Subtle Energy Techniques
CYNDI DALE

Renowned author Cyndi Dale invites you into the world of subtle energy, where you'll explore auras, chakras, intuition, and the basics of her groundbreaking energy techniques. Whether your goals are physical, psychological, or spiritual, these methods can help you achieve your desires, heal your wounds, and live an enlightened life.

978-0-7387-5161-0, 288 pp., 5 x 7   **$14.99**

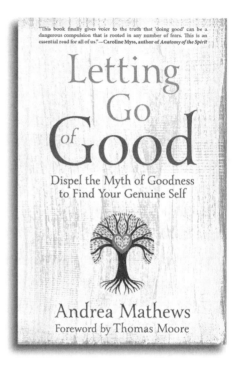

"This book finally gives voice to the truth that 'doing good' can be a dangerous compulsion that is rooted in any number of fears. This is an essential read for all of us."—Caroline Myss, author of *Anatomy of the Spirit*

Letting
Go
of Good

Dispel the Myth of Goodness
to Find Your Genuine Self

Andrea Mathews
Foreword by Thomas Moore

Letting Go of Good
Dispel the Myth of Goodness to Find Your Genuine Self
ANDREA MATHEWS

Rediscover your true self with *Letting Go of Good*, an empowering guide to dismantling the false connection between being good and being worthy. While exposing the dangers of the guilt-led life, practicing psychotherapist Andrea Mathews shares innovative tools and techniques for healing, including how to understand and dialogue with emotions, develop intuition and discernment, and make decisions from a place of honest desire and compassion.

Featuring a foreword by Thomas Moore, author of *Care of the Soul*, this book provides the guidance you need to embrace the real, authentic you. With illuminating composite examples from Andrea's clinical experience and a powerful exploration of the pathway to healing, *Letting Go of Good* presents a breakthrough approach to creating genuine relationships and awakening your true self to find peace.

978-0-7387-5223-5, 288 pp., 6 x 9   **$17.99**

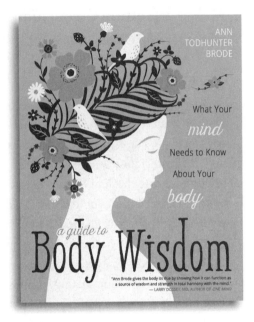

ANN
TODHUNTER
BRODE

What Your
mind
Needs to Know
About Your
body

a guide to
Body Wisdom

"Ann Brode gives the body its due by showing how it can function as
a source of wisdom and strength in total harmony with the mind."
— LARRY DOSSEY, MD, AUTHOR OF *ONE MIND*

A Guide to Body Wisdom
What Your Mind Needs to Know About Your Body
Ann Todhunter Brode

Deepen your spirituality, heal old wounds, and enhance your emotional and physical wellness by engaging in a conversation with your body. This innovative, down-to-earth guide teaches you how to listen to, understand, and work with your body's innate wisdom in everyday living.

A Guide to Body Wisdom provides step-by-step instruction on how to create a personalized self-care regimen that works. You'll learn to quiet your mind and live consciously in your body through a variety of practices, including breathwork, mindful eating, meditation, affirmation, and positive habit building. Featuring simple exercises and techniques, as well as a Body IQ quiz, this valuable book helps you end negative thinking, develop intuition, improve relationships, boost creativity and personal power, and much more.

978-0-7387-5695-0, 288 pp., 7½ x 9¼   **$21.99**

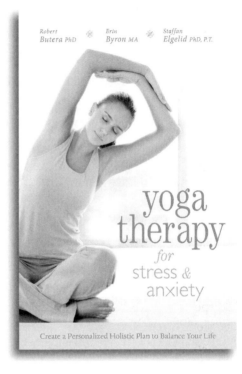

Yoga Therapy for Stress & Anxiety
Create a Personalized Holistic Plan to Balance Your Life
Robert Butera, PhD
Erin Byron, MA
Staffan Elgelid, PhD

Create a personalized path to healing with this step-by-step guide to holistic change. Comprehensive and accessible no matter your skill level, *Yoga Therapy for Stress & Anxiety* helps you understand what creates a stress-filled life so that you may choose a life of ease instead. Through yoga practice and the lesser-known lifestyle aspects of yoga, you will be able to face all situations from the calm perspective of the higher self.

Incorporating exercises, breathing techniques, meditation, and many other tools, this guide provides effective methods for repairing areas of imbalance and identifying your needs. Learn about the five yogic paths of psychology, intellect, health, work, and relationships. Apply a variety of yoga postures for relaxation, improved attitude and sleep, self-acceptance, and more. With the transformative power of a whole-lifestyle approach, you will achieve wellness in your mind, body, and soul.

978-0-7387-4575-6, 360 pp., 6 x 9 $19.99

To order, call 1-877-NEW-WRLD or visit llewellyn.com
Prices subject to change without notice

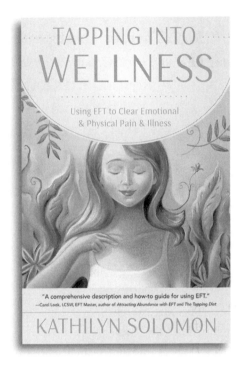

TAPPING INTO
WELLNESS

Using EFT to Clear Emotional
& Physical Pain & Illness

"A comprehensive description and how-to guide for using EFT."
—Carol Look, LCSW, EFT Master, author of *Attracting Abundance with EFT* and *The Tapping Diet*

KATHILYN SOLOMON

Tapping Into Wellness
Using EFT to Clear Emotional & Physical Pain & Illness
Kathilyn Solomon

Imagine experiencing vibrant health, peace, abundance, and optimism every day. *Tapping Into Wellness* shares an innovative tool called Emotional Freedom Technique (EFT), which allows you to have all this and more, literally at your fingertips. Join Kathilyn Solomon as she shares simple instructions, powerful and practical exercises, and real-life case studies from this world of miracles.

EFT (also known as tapping) is a fast-spreading, easy-to-learn, and effective approach for men, women, children, and animals. This guide draws on the latest EFT Gold Standard, showing you how to work through physical or emotional problems and challenges. Often referred to as acupuncture without needles, tapping can help you:

- Resolve chronic pain and illness, cravings, and addictions
- Overcome stress, anxiety, and phobias
- Activate your body's own natural healing system
- Gain relief from haunting memories and trauma
- Experience resilience, positive energy, and improved health

978-0-7387-3788-1, 336 pp., 6 x 9　　　　　　　　**$19.99**

To order, call 1-877-NEW-WRLD or visit llewellyn.com
Prices subject to change without notice

DELLA TEMPLE

Tame
Your
Inner
Critic

※

Find Peace & Contentment
to Live Your Life
on Purpose

Tame Your Inner Critic

Find Peace & Contentment to Live Your Life on Purpose

DELLA TEMPLE

Uncover the authentic you, control the critic within, and find the peace you need to live your life on purpose. Learn to silence the persistent chatter of your inner critic and replace it with the voice of your inner guidance, your spirit.

Tame Your Inner Critic takes you on a journey of self-discovery, exploring the energy of your thoughts and turning the negative into positive. Discover how to use your innate intuitive abilities to heal these energies and discard judgments and criticisms that have built up over the years. Find your true north—your own internal wisdom that is connected to the divine and gives you guidance. With specialized exercises and meditations, this book shows you how to banish negativity, improve your relationships, and realize new ways to share your gifts with the world around you.

978-0-7387-4395-0, 264 pp., 5 ¼ x 8   **$15.99**

The
Body
Heals
Itself

How *Deeper Awareness* of Your *Muscles* and Their *Emotional Connection* Can *Help You Heal*

EMILY A. FRANCIS

The Body Heals Itself

*How Deeper Awareness of Your Muscles and Their
Emotional Connection Can Help You Heal*

Emily A. Francis

You know a lot about the emotions in your mind and heart, but you probably don't know much about the emotions in your muscle body. The muscles are storehouses of emotion, and pain in those muscles is how your body reveals what needs to be healed—both emotionally and physically. Organized by muscle groups, *The Body Heals Itself* is your ideal guide to understanding the link between your emotions and muscle bodies.

This book acts as a road map for the energetic journey within your own body, showing you how to recognize and release stored emotions to let go of pain. You'll discover which emotions are often paired with a specific muscle area and how muscles speak of everything from past traumas to current celebrations. Using stretches, affirmations, visualizations, and more, Emily A. Francis teaches you to unite your mind and body for better health and emotional well-being.

978-0-7387-5073-6, 312 pp., 7½ x 9¼   **$21.99**

KAVITHA CHINNAIYAN, MD

"A must-read for anyone who wants to truly understand what it means to
live whole-heartedly—regardless of one's state of health."
—Christiane Northrup, MD, *New York Times* bestselling author of *Goddesses Never Age*

The
Heart of
Wellness

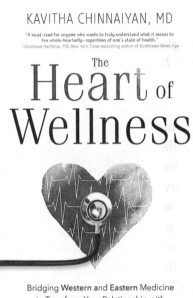

Bridging **Western** and **Eastern** Medicine
to Transform Your Relationship with
Habits, Lifestyle, and Health

The Heart of Wellness

Bridging Western and Eastern Medicine to Transform Your Relationship with Habits, Lifestyle, and Health

KAVITHA M. CHINNAIYAN, MD

Transform your relationship with habits, lifestyle, and disease using Dr. Kavitha Chinnaiyan's remarkable approach to health. Integrating modern medicine and the ancient wisdom of Yoga, Vedanta, and Ayurveda, *The Heart of Wellness* shows you how to break free of the false assumption that disease is something you need to fight. Instead, you'll explore the mind-body connection and your true nature so that you can end suffering and embrace the unlimited bliss of who you are.

You'll begin by examining the nature of disease: the causative and risk factors, the role of diet, exercise, and medication, and how Eastern and Western medical practices can come together. A holistic and self-paced practice is outlined, based on the author's successful Heal Your Heart Free Your Soul program. With it you'll learn to reduce stress, attend to inner needs with meditation and breathwork, declutter your outer life, increase forgiveness and gratitude, and so much more.

978-0-7387-5199-3, 288 pp., 6 x 9 **$19.99**

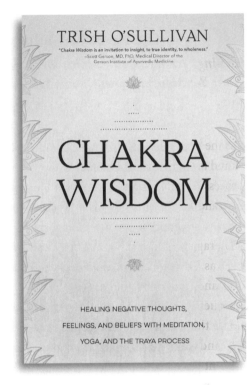

TRISH O'SULLIVAN

"*Chakra Wisdom* is an invitation to insight, to true identity, to wholeness."
—Scott Gerson, MD, PhD, Medical Director of the
Gerson Institute of Ayurvedic Medicine

CHAKRA
WISDOM

HEALING NEGATIVE THOUGHTS,

FEELINGS, AND BELIEFS WITH MEDITATION,

YOGA, AND THE TRAYA PROCESS

Chakra Wisdom

Healing Negative Thoughts, Feelings, and Beliefs with Meditation, Yoga, and the Traya Process

Trish O'Sullivan

Just as the body is able to heal itself, nature has provided a way for the mind to heal as well. In *Chakra Wisdom*, you will discover how to process emotional and spiritual blocks as you release negative energy and heal the wounds that interfere with personal fulfillment.

Therapist, yogi, and healer Trish O'Sullivan shares a system known as Traya, which utilizes the chakras as tools to better understand, work with, and heal the mind. This process includes techniques for connecting to your inner teacher and the deep mind so that you can recover from illness and trauma, reduce stress, and enter the stream of healing energy. By combining consistent practice, work with the higher self, and insights from Western psychotherapy, this book invites you to cultivate your spirit and realize the full potential of your life.

978-0-7387-5743-8, 288 pp., 6 x 9   **17.99**
